HOLISTIC HEALTH

*The Truth About Wellness
And Prevention*

DR. ERIC JASZEWSKI, DC

Important Information For the Reader

This information presented in this book has been compiled from my experience and research. It is offered as a view of the relationship between healthy living, exercise, balance, and health. This book is not intended for self-diagnosis or treatment of disease, nor is it a substitute for the advice and care of a licensed health care provider. Sharing of the information in this book with the attending physician is highly desirable.

This book is intended solely to help you make better judgements concerning your long-term health goals. If you are experiencing health problems, you should consult a qualified physician immediately. Remember early examination and detection are important to successful treatment of all diseases.

DEDICATION

To my wife Jenna and our kids...

Brooke, Autumn, Bryce, Aubrey, Brayden, Blayke, Bria, Asher & Axel...

Thank you all for loving me and for giving me a reason...

You are all my reasons!

TABLE OF CONTENTS

INTRODUCTION 1

CHAPTER 1: Where United States Ranks in Quality of Healthcare 10

CHAPTER 2: What Is "Health"? 27

CHAPTER 3: The Health Model vs. The Sick Model 40

CHAPTER 4: The Germ Theory Debunked 54

CHAPTER 5: The Importance Of Epigenetics 69

CHAPTER 6: Wellness and Prevention 82

CHAPTER 7: The Nervous System Central to Good Health 92

CHAPTER 8: The Spine 99

CHAPTER 9: The Mistakes We Make Everyday 105

CHAPTER 10: The Pierce Results System & Specific Chiropractic Adjustments 117

CHAPTER 11: Diagnostic Methods Used in Chiropractic 122

CHAPTER 12: Phases Of Healing 127

CHAPTER 13: Spinal Degeneration 138

CHAPTER 14: Scoliosis 156

CHAPTER 15: Text Neck 169

CHAPTER 16: Perfect Posture 180

CHAPTER 17: The Benefits Of Prenatal Chiropractic 188

CHAPTER 18: Chiropractic for Life 202

INTRODUCTION

This is a book about chiropractic. There are many questions about the origins of chiropractic, and how it is utilized today, along with how it is viewed by the mainstream medical field and traditional medicine. That is one of the purposes of this book.

Another reason why I wanted to write a book on chiropractic was to give both my patients and those who may be skeptical about how chiropractic works a look at the logic behind this science. Yes, it is a science and a precise one at that. As more medical doctors come to realize the benefits of proper chiropractic care they too may find themselves referring patients they once thought could only be treated by prescription drugs and surgery to the non-evasive, gentle care of their local chiropractor.

In researching this book, I sought out the experience of other chiropractors so that I could add their research and expertise to my own in creating a well-rounded publication that would inform and educate my readers not only on chiropractic, but also on how to live a life centered in wellness. Much to my surprise, there are not too many others who have written such a common sense and down to earth guide to chiropractic. We have our textbooks and clinical trial summaries, but not a whole lot out there for the average person.

This gave great purpose to my publication. I wanted a sensible summary of various medical conditions and lifestyle choices that can help you better understand the chiropractic way of life.

The larger scope of this book is to educate and inform readers about the part chiropractic plays in a life of good physical health and wellness. It takes the approach that chiropractic, along with other lifestyle choices and good habits, can create a sense of wellness that goes beyond fighting disease and illness.

Good health and high spirits go hand in hand. When you understand how each activity you participate in, every action you take to feed and nourish your body and mind, and how you react to external factors, you will also gain some insight into how to be truly "well" in every sense of the word.

So, what can you expect from this book? Common sense! We as a culture are so inundated with thinking that, in order for something to work, it has to be complicated. Nothing could be further from the truth. If it's complicated it won't be used. It's that simple.

Look at the personal computer revolution. Up until the introduction of the Apple computer, computers were feared, and no one used them - not the masses at least. Then along came Steve Jobs, who revolutionized the personal computer industry through simplicity. It is time to revolutionize the health industry by creating concepts that are easy to understand and most importantly, are applied because simplicity is the key. If it's not simple you will have all the excuses in the world to not use them.

Keeping the concept of simplicity in mind, this book is going to talk about things that are simple to do that can make a huge difference in your overall health. Goals and accomplishments must be perceived as being doable or we aren't going to even attempt them. The processes discussed in this book will be full of easy, doable processes that can make a world of a difference in your life.

We unfortunately believe that we can change our lives overnight. The truth is that we can change our *mind* overnight, but our body doesn't change that quickly. This is because whatever it was that created the condition of our body didn't happen overnight or even take one or two weeks; it took a lifetime. So if you want to change your health for good, you must look at the healing factor differently. Look at it as an ongoing process that you begin today.

What you need to do to get something out of this book is begin by opening your mind. They say the mind is like a parachute, and it won't work if it's not opened. You must have an open mind to try out new ideas, especially those actions that may not be as widely accepted by the mainstream population.

We as a society fear change. Yet we continue on the path that has brought us to the condition of health that we now experience. Somehow we expect that staying on the same path can yield a different result, than the last time we started down it. Curiosity might very well be the help you need to bridge the gap from where you are to where you want to be. Be curious with trying new things. Don't have mental atherosclerosis. Don't have hardening of the mental arteries. Be open to new possibilities. Be open to doing something and it not "working at first." That's okay. You'll just try again.

It is funny that, as a society, we tend to believe that in order for us to be successful, we must succeed at something on the first try. That is simply just a myth. It doesn't exist; it's not possible for that to be true. For that myth to be true, we would have to know exactly what was going to happen and purposely do the wrong thing. If that were the case, then at that point I would call it a mistake. It is a mistake, then, because we knew better.

Life is a process. It is an experience. We must go through life with the courage that we will sometimes fall or sometimes fail. But so what! All we do is just get back up. That is the key to success: to get back up when you fall.

Open your heart and open your mind and begin to explore the possibilities of a new life. The life I am talking about is a life with more energy, more vitality, and most of all, a life full of HEALTH!

Stumbling Blocks To Success

Fear can be one of the biggest obstacles that can prevent you from getting anything from this book. Fear rids you of any desire, and justifies why you continue to do what you already do. Don't let fear hold you back. It can rob you of your dreams, and it can certainly drain you of your health and well-being.

Excuses will dry up your motivation more than anything out there. Don't make any more excuses. There is a saying, "It's not the situation that you are in that holds you back; it is the excuses that you use to justify the situation." Don't let excuses come in the way of you implementing what you learn from this book. Grab some strategies and go with them. See for yourself what they can do for you. The bottom line is to decide what you want.

Many people tell me as a doctor, "I'm tired of feeling this; I don't want to feel pain anymore." Or they may tell me, "I don't want to feel tired anymore." They tell me what they *don't* want to feel, and I explain to them, "If you are so concerned with what you don't want to feel, how can you concentrate on what you *do* want?" So, focus on what you want, not on what you don't want. That is the key!

It is my hope that by reading this book you too can come to the decision that chiropractic care is a part of health care and wellness that everyone needs - not just those with back problems. It can provide you with a proactive approach to your health. It can also open the body up to its full self-healing potential. Not too many doctors and pharmacists would dare make that claim. I invite you to read on and learn more about this proven scientific method of wellness and all that chiropractic encompasses.

The Simplicity Philosophy

Bottom line to good heath and a system of managing it that you can use for a lifetime is simplicity. You must grab on to things that can work. Simple plans work. Amazing results await you as you read ahead. All you need is the confidence in yourself to implement the following information. Then you will find yourself making huge gains within your health.

Phenomenal healing powers are within you waiting to be unleashed. The key is to focus on the wins, and not get distracted by the setbacks. You will get them; we all will. It is not being negative by saying this. It is being real.

All of the principles you are going to learn in this book are based on laws of nature. They are not some kind of magical, cool-sounding approach that contradicts simple common sense. They are quite simply the laws of life or, perhaps, you could think of them as laws of nature.

What you arc going to learn here are the same principles that farmers abide by. They call it "The law of the farm." Basically, it is a natural law that affects us all, but too many people live by the effect of this law, rather than rule over it. They let what happens control them, instead of controlling what happens. You must understand that there are many theories out there and many have strong merit. But what good are they if you don't take action and are not consistent?

One example is the yo-yo weight loss and gain cycle which results from diet fads in this country. It alone is creating such a level of disease that it's driving health care costs through the roof. We must change something now!

Technology's Role in Health Care

Sure, technology has had a great impact on healthcare. We see the evolution of the x-ray and ultrasound that lets us see into the body what we could only approximate before. In this book, however, you will learn about a technology that is so simple to use that it will blow you away. You see that health should not be complicated. Anyone trying to complicate health is trying to get you to be dependent on them, so you rely on them solely, and forget your own judgment.

That has been the problem within the medical profession for some time. We have abided by the opinions of our healthcare professionals and their latest technologies, but it has brought us no more health than we expected. As a matter of fact, we in the United States fail miserably as a society according to the World Health Organization (WHO).

The WHO reports that the U.S. ranks 37th out of 200 countries in terms of quality of individual health and wellness. To put that into perspective, Columbia is ranked

39th. How can we accept such mediocre results from a country that spends more dollars on health care than any other country in the world?

What we are doing is simply not working. Innovation is at the heart of this book. No more complex strategies; we are going to get to the simple, bare bones concepts that you can immediately use in your everyday life and that can truly make a difference in your life.

Break away from the old and decide today for yourself that you are going to use a technology that will truly make a difference in your life. You deserve it, and those around you deserve someone who comes to the table alive, refreshed, energetic, and not just a partial representation of themselves. You deserve to reach the full you at your greatest potential! It should not be an option; this is your birthright.

Why do we need to think outside the box? This expression has been used for many years now and although it sounds cliché, it holds true more today than ever. We must change our paradigm from disease care, which we are clearly in, to a preventative care way of looking at health. It's the most cost-effective way of taking care of our bodies.

This is not a new concept in other areas, so why should it be so under utilized when it comes to health? The automotive companies have known about it since cars were invented. They are well aware that if you give your car preventative care such as periodic tune ups and oil changes they will last longer. It's that simple.

So, the key is to trim the fat from our health care. I believe the best way to do that is not to rely on symptoms. If you wait until there are symptoms, most often you are too late. You will learn more about this later in the book, but please keep that concept in mind.

The tests and processes we are using to determine health are not showing the consequences of our diets of ten years ago. It doesn't show what is going on with our arteries from the standpoint of what the food we consume today is going to do to our arteries 5 or 10 years from now. Insanity has crippled this health care system, and we must do something about this now, before it's too late.

If we continue at this rate in 50 years we have the unfortunate opportunity of bankrupting this country due to health care costs. Costs have gone through the roof for HMO's and other insurance plans, and it is predicted that within 5 – 10 years health care deductibles will reach an annual level of more than $5,000 per person. That is ridiculous.

You can do your part to change this. We all can when we approach our own health and that of our families in a preventative, proactive manner.

CHAPTER 1

WHERE UNITED STATES RANKS IN QUALITY OF HEALTHCARE

Until the early 1990s, there was considerable disagreement amongst gerontologists and demographers regarding what the future might bring despite certain high-income countries having achieved significant improvement in life expectancy. On one hand pessimists believed that deaths beyond the age of eighty were due to issues associated with senescence and intractable aging processes.

It was commonly believed that without any major breakthroughs in terms of biomedical interventions, it would be highly unlikely for the average life expectancy to significantly increase past the age of eighty-five. However, some optimists argued that there was still potential for further improvements in longevity; they thought that existing population estimates were too conservative and did not take all factors into consideration.

Demographers have had difficulty studying patterns of mortality and morbidity at advanced ages because of limited, unreliable and non-comparable data sources on an international level. This is particularly the case in the United States, where demographers have traditionally been wary of relying on mortality data related to older generations, due to doubts about the accuracy or validity of such data obtained from the census. For years, it has been well known that many Americans tend to be overweight and lead a sedentary lifestyle. Unfortunately, despite being one of the most expensive healthcare systems in the world, we often produce results that are less than optimal. The life expectancy in the United States has also been observed to be lesser than in other wealthy countries; and the infant mortality rates far higher than those seen in other nations.

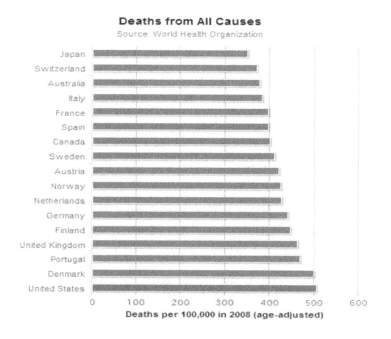

A panel of doctors, epidemiologists, demographers and other researchers was commissioned by the National Research Council and the Institute of Medicine, to better comprehend the health disparities among Americans, compared to citizens from 16 other countries such as Australia, Japan, Canada and nations found in Western Europe. The team gathered publicly accessible data from organizations such as the World Health Organization, and the Organization for Economic Cooperation and Development.

The research results were shocking, to say the least! They uncovered a consistent and extensive pattern of poor health in U.S. citizens, from infancy to adulthood. Compared to other developed countries, Americans were more prone to fatalities resulting from injuries, homicides, alcohol and drug abuse. Furthermore, our nation had some of the highest rates of heart disease, lung disease, obesity and diabetes in the world. The researchers involved in this study concluded that while America was once portrayed as a beacon of health and wellness, its current state suggests that it is losing ground in those exact areas.

For the past three decades, Americans - particularly men - have had one of the lowest chances in living past the age of 50. The major contributing factors to this devastating statistic are homicides, car accidents, other types of accidents. As well as non-communicable diseases, such as diabetes and heart disease, and perinatal problems like low birth weights and premature births that leads to a high infant mortality rates.

Among the most striking report findings between the studies countries, were these from the US:

- The US has some of the world's highest rates of death by violence.
- We have the highest death rate due to car accidents.
- The highest chance of child death, before the age of five.
- The second-highest death rate due to coronary heart disease.
- The second-highest death rate caused by lung disease.
- The highest teen pregnancy rate.
- The highest rate of women dying, due to complications related to pregnancy and childbirth (the maternal death rate).

Today, Americans are presented with a brighter outlook when it comes to surviving cancer or even suffering a stroke. For those who make it to the age of 75, it is likely that they will outlive many others of their generation. Nevertheless, these encouraging findings cannot be seen as an indication that all is well in terms of personal and public health. Far from it, there are an array of issues that diminish this relatively optimistic outlook.

Where Does U.S. Rank In Crisis Care Intervention?

For well over a century, American presidents have been trying to find an appropriate way to provide healthcare coverage for everyone, that is both widely available and not run by the government. Through this entire period, balancing the demands of public interest with private influence as well as meeting the needs of diverse stakeholders has proven to be a tough task to achieve.

The American healthcare system is also very complex and fragmented, with different states having their own individual policies on healthcare coverage. This adds an additional layer of complexity to an already complex problem of providing affordable healthcare to all citizens.

According to the World Health Report 2000, which focused on improving performance in healthcare systems, the United States ranked as having the 37th best healthcare system, on a global level. This has been widely discussed and debated in light of current reform initiatives concerning our healthcare.

Despite the fact that the United States has one of the most expensive healthcare systems in the world, it still ranks last out of eleven other industrialized countries when it comes to measures of health system quality, efficiency, access to care, and equity according to a new Commonwealth Fund report. These countries include Australia, Canada, France, Germany, the Netherlands, New Zealand, Norway, Sweden, Switzerland and the

United Kingdom. Although all of these countries have room for improvement in their healthcare systems, too, the U.S. stands out as having both the *highest* healthcare costs, *and* the lowest performance. In 2011 alone, the total health expenditures per person in the U.S. amounted to $8,508, compared to the $3,406 spent in the United Kingdom (who ranked first in their overall quality of healthcare).

Despite claims from some that international comparisons are not helpful, due to the uniqueness of the United States, rankings play an important role in numerous areas. In 2006, the U.S. ranked first in terms of healthcare spending per capita, yet it placed 39th in infant mortality, 43rd for adult female mortality, 42nd for adult male mortality, and 36th in life expectancy.

These rankings have sparked a flurry of discussion among academics, the government, and the general public, as they ask why we are spending so much, yet achieving so little in terms of health outcomes. Further research is needed to determine if there are certain factors that explain why the U.S. is not seeing better health outcomes despite its high healthcare spending, compared to other countries.

The current proposals for healthcare reforms in the United States focus almost exclusively on expanding insurance coverage, reducing the rate of costs through increased efficiencies, and investing in preventive care and wellness programs. These efforts are aimed at protecting households against unnecessary financial hardship and could potentially save from 18,000 to 44,000 lives each year. Although the United States has been struggling to keep up with other high-income countries when it comes to health outcomes, there are numerous approaches that can be taken to try and close this gap, or even just slow down its decline in the rankings, than just expanding insurance coverage.

Dr. Ralph Snyderman, MD and Chancellor Emeritus at the Duke University School of Medicine, has stated that the current healthcare system in the United States is more reactive than preventive; it waits to address symptoms of disease until they arise, rather than invest time and effort into preventing them from occurring in the first place. This has been echoed by Dr. Ka-Kit Hui, MD from the UCLA Center for East-West Medicine, and the Wallis Annenberg Professor in Integrative East-West Medicine, who believes that healthcare should spend more time focused on prevention.

The idea of preventative health care is gaining traction among medical experts, and services are now beginning to be provided by doctors and hospitals to help keep Americans healthier.

In light of the current situation where healthcare reforms have been pushed back, it is important to consider how our healthcare system should be reformed as we move forward. As it currently stands the system that we refer to as 'healthcare' is predominantly a 'disease-care' system, which focuses on treating existing diseases and illnesses with medications and surgeries.

At medical school, the education of medical doctors generally focuses on addressing symptoms of disease rather than learning how to prevent them. While a healthy diet is critical for maintaining good health, medical students receive limited instruction on nutrition and other lifestyle changes which can help keep people healthy, such as exercise and relaxation therapies. Moreover, their training does not provide much information on alternative therapies which have been used by different cultures for centuries to heal and maintain good health.

Modern Western medicine and science have made remarkable advances over several decades, vastly improving the lives of countless people. From trauma and burns, to emergency medical and surgical treatments, the advancements made have been nothing short of miraculous.

Through modern drugs many illnesses can be treated effectively, and be efficiently managed, when used correctly. In addition, medical technology has advanced to the point where even complex illnesses, such as cancer and heart disease can be managed with a variety of therapeutic options.

In an ideal healthcare system, modern western medicine would be employed in a way that maximizes its potential benefits. This could include crisis care, acute medical and surgical emergency care, and other scenarios where it can be the most suitable form of treatment. At the same time, natural remedies that are non-toxic, and non-invasive, should take precedence whenever possible. When it comes to preventing and treating chronic diseases, the most effective approach is to adopt a healthy lifestyle that includes a balanced diet, physical activity, stress management, and other benign approaches.

When Did Big Pharma Take Over?

The global pharmaceutical industry is oftentimes referred to as "Big Pharma", a term which has been marked by a sense of demonization within recent years. Steve Novella, an MD and academic clinical neurologist at Yale University School of Medicine, states that the term is used as a shorthand for all the various agencies involved in the trillion-dollar "prescription pharmaceutical pie" - including corporations, regulators, NGOs, politicians and physicians. Through this context, author Robert Blaskiewicz notes that conspiracy theorists have often used the term to represent a cast of villains, working together in pursuit of their own financial gain and influence.

Thus, "Big Pharma" is the pejorative nickname often given to the pharmaceutical industry. Critics of the industry tend to utilize this nickname when debating on some the following issues:

- That various pharmaceutical companies to some people seem to look for ways to capitalize on the misfortune of the ill, injured, or dying, for monetary gain. They are claimed to invent new kinds of maladies, diseases, or afflictions to drive up the

demand for their products and drugs; instead of producing better medications which could help more people become healthy. This can lead to the creation of drugs that can be highly addictive, as well as create dependency problems for those using them.
- Critics claim that, rather than censoring cheaper or more effective alternative treatments, it is important to support measures that are considered effective, but which have fewer or no side-effects, and which are less damaging.

As families and patients around the world become increasingly more vocal about their dissatisfaction with "Big Pharma", a growing number of criticisms are being raised. Many are alarmed by the prevalence of medications that not only seem to fail to cure or prevent disease, but which also seem to cause more harm than good, and lead to serious side effects or dependence issues.

When Did Insurance Companies Come About?

The history of insurance is a rich and varied one, tracing its roots back to the creation of modern insurance practices in order to protect against different kinds of risks. In particular, this includes cargo, property damage or destruction, and death due to accidents or medical malpractice. Insurance companies aim to provide long-term financial stability for both the public and private sectors.

In the United States, health insurance refers to any program which helps cover or subsidize the cost of medical expenses, both through private policies and those funded by the government. Common synonyms for this type of coverage include "health coverage," "healthcare coverage" and "health benefits." In a more technical sense, this term can describe any type of insurance which helps to pay for medical services, including both private policies and public programs.

Private insurance plans are typically purchased by individuals or employers, to help cover the cost of medical care. Major medical expenses can be spread across an entire population through these plans, reducing the risk that an individual will face expensive bills on their own, in the event of a serious illness or accident.

Health insurance can refer to a variety of coverages, including medical expenses and disability care. In addition, it may also provide protection for long-term nursing or custodial care services, depending on the type of plan that is chosen. Unfortunately, research has shown that over 40% of those insured are unsatisfied with their coverage, indicating that their plans do not meet their needs, as of 2007.

Insurance was quite a late addition to the American healthcare system, primarily due to the number of known risks, as well as an undefined number of unknown ones. Eventually, it did gain popularity, partly thanks to one of the most well-known figures in American history. In 1752, Benjamin Franklin made an addition to his many enterprises by becoming an insurer. This was the same year that saw the foundation of the Philadelphia Contributionship for the Insurance of Houses from Loss by Fire, which was America's first mutual fire insurance company. During this time, buildings were mostly constructed using wood as a primary material, and homes were built in close proximity to one another. This was initially done for security reasons, but as cities expanded developers wanted to maximize use of their land by building as many homes on any one plot as possible.

In today's world, the internet has revolutionized the insurance industry by expanding its reach. Customers now have more options than ever before, with the ability to search online for the best rates and coverage. Companies are also taking advantage of this global market, merging with other financial service providers to increase their size and broaden their services. This integration of services allows companies to offer their customers convenience and value, rather than just focusing on price.

In recent years, the number of Americans without health insurance has been drastically reduced, largely due to the implementation of reforms outlined in the Affordable Care Act of 2010. Yet, despite these changes, the rate of growth in healthcare costs remains consistently high. In fact, national health expenditures are estimated to rise by 4.7% per person, per year, from 2016 to 2025.

Public healthcare spending is another area of concern; it accounted for 29% of the federal mandated spending in 1990, and 35% of it in 2000.

How Are Medicare And Medicaid Funded?

Medicare is a federal health insurance program that provides coverage for individuals aged 65 and older, as well as people suffering with disabilities, regardless of their income level. It is estimated that this system offers protection to around 58 million individuals across the United States. Each state is given the responsibility of setting their own eligibility requirements, as well as the scope of services that they offer. Additionally, each state has the power to set their own payment rates for services and to administer their own individual Medicaid program.

To ensure that these programs are working properly, the Centers for Medicare and Medicaid Services (CMS) of the Department of Health and Human Services (HHS) oversees both Medicare and Medicaid.

The Medicare program, which was established in 1965, provides senior citizens with health insurance coverage that is comparable to the protection available for non-elderly and non-disabled Americans in the private sector. This includes hospital insurance (Part A), supplementary insurance (Part B), which covers outpatient and home health services, as well as physician visits and prescription drug coverage (Part D). Seniors also have the option of enrolling in private plans (Part C), called Medicare Advantage, to cover their services.

The Medicare program currently covers 44 million people, 37 million seniors and 7 million disabled Americans. It is financed through Federal payroll taxes, general tax revenues, and beneficiary premiums.

The Medicaid program is a joint effort between the federal government and all the individual states. The Federal Medical Assistance Percentage (FMAP) – which is set by the federal government – dictates how much each state must contribute to their own Medicaid expenditures, to fund care and services that are available under their state plan. Each state can also establish their own Medicaid provider payment rates within federal guidelines, which can be paid through either fee-for-service or managed care arrangements. To alter their payment rate policies, states must submit a State Plan Amendment (SPA) to the Centers for Medicare and Medicaid Services (CMS) for review and approval.

Why Can't We Buy Health Insurance Like We Can Buy Auto Insurance?

Imagine what it might be like if automobile insurance covered all the expenses related to owning a car - from routine oil changes, engine maintenance, to worn-out tires and brakes, rust damage, and more. It is easy to see how the cost of such a policy could skyrocket! This is the current reality of our healthcare: as plans increasingly cover more services and procedures, the costs of coverage continue to rise. Insurance companies are paying for far more than earlier, in response to consumer demand and state mandates.

The demand for greater access to healthcare benefits is becoming more and more pronounced, with many considering it a personal right to have every available medical service at their disposal.

Unfortunately, the costs associated with these additional benefits are often not clear to consumers, leading them to believe that they are getting something "for free". To meet this demand, health plans may choose to expand coverage on their own or be forced by politicians to do so.

To make healthcare more affordable, state governments should stop mandating additional benefits and instead focus on providing essential services at a manageable cost. Private insurance companies and government programs, like Medicare, should also agree to provide only those medical treatments that are both cost-effective and necessary.

Insurance is designed to pool people's money together, to provide coverage for expenses that are substantial and often unexpected. It's meant to be a safeguard for when calamitous events take place. By taking on more of their healthcare costs Americans may have the incentive needed to develop healthier habits, such as exercising regularly, eating nutritious food, and refraining from smoking and excessive drinking. Consequently, this would result in a healthier population which would lead to fewer medical services being necessary, and lower healthcare costs and premiums.

Overall, insurance is a valuable tool for protecting people against losses that can't be reasonably anticipated or controlled. By providing coverage for such events, it can help to safeguard individuals, families, and businesses from financial disaster. It can also incentivize individuals to pursue healthier lifestyles, ultimately resulting in lower costs for the entire population. By transforming healthcare insurance into a system which only covers essential services and procedures, more Americans would be able to obtain coverage and the number of uninsured individuals in the US would be drastically reduced.

Why Don't Insurance Companies Reward The Health Conscious?

Life insurance is a common concern for families, given the number of options and rates available. The cost of an individual life insurance plan usually depends on a variety of factors, including elements that are out of the person's control, such as hereditary health issues. Other determining factors include age, their medical history and personal lifestyle habits.

As one of the major stakeholders in healthcare reform, insurance companies are actively working to reduce costs. Studies have shown that about 50% of medical expenses can be attributed to a handful of chronic conditions, such as conditions related to obesity, high blood pressure, high cholesterol, and diabetes. To address this issue, insurers are investing in disease management programs which help people with chronic conditions lead healthier lifestyles and reduce the cost of long-term medical care. As the costs of healthcare continue to rise and changes to payment processing systems come about slowly, insurers have been exploring various ways to incentivize their members to take control of their health. These patient engagement programs range from small monetary rewards to extensive wellness coaching systems. It remains to be seen how effective these initiatives will be in the long run, yet many in the industry are determined to find out.

CHAPTER 2

WHAT IS "HEALTH"?

If I were to ask you to define the term "health," what kind of answer would you give me? There is a general opinion and consensus that good health (1) can be feeling "fine," (2) is when everything is working okay, or (3) when pain is absent.

All these definitions are partial and far from being complete. Taber's Medical Dictionary defines health as "a condition in which all body and mind functions are normally active". The World Health Organization defines health as "complete physical, mental, or social well-being", rather than merely the absence of disease or infirmity. So, the next question to ask is: How does one quantify health? In a sense, health is equal to balance. How do we determine balance? What are the determining factors in the balancing equation? To answer this, we must first ask: What comprises the overall health scheme? Also, what broad gauge can be used to reflect on the quality of health we experience, or the lack thereof?

To get to the core of good health, you must start at the cellular level; the balancing act begins there. The quality of your life is based on the quality of the life of your cells, as you are comprised of over 70 trillion cells. When these cells work optimally and in perfect harmony, you will have health; but how does one quantify this?

Now, if health equals balance, we can state that the opposite of health is not a disease, but rather a "dis-ease"; meaning a lack of balance or ease. It can also be said that this would then be when the cells are not functioning correctly. Raymond Francis, a chemist and graduate of MIT, found through his research and believes that there is only one reason why any disease is created. That reason is simply due to cells not functioning correctly. When you think about that statement, it makes sense.

Now, there are only two reasons why cells do not work appropriately: they are the following:

- The cells are not receiving proper nutrition.
- The cells are not eliminating the waste produced by the cell's normal processes.

Now, there are many reasons why cells can become dysfunctional. Those reasons are as follows:

- Lack of appropriate levels of oxygen.
- Lack of nutrients.
- The inability to eliminate waste.
- Improper nerve impulses to the cell.

By gaining a thorough understanding of this process, we can review the multiple stages of health. From birth, every person is born with an innate capacity to experience optimal well-being; however, if there is any disruption in the connection between your nervous system and body systems – you will be unable to access or maintain good health.

Years pass us by, and our cells begin to alter, before we feel the actual effects of ageing. Eventually, our bodies transition from a state of cellular creation — anabolic metabolism — to one where more cells die than are replaced; catabolic metabolism. To reduce the speed at which this occurs, it is paramount that we do all that we can to decelerate this process as much as possible!

To be familiar with the complexity of health, it is important to know and comprehend its different stages. The first stage is ideal wellness where all parts are integrated harmoniously as they were originally intended. Sadly, over time, due to various psychological and physiological pressures, we start a downward spiral into imbalance or more accurately referred to as "dis-ease". This signals that something needs our attention in our bodies, and our lives. Health can quickly be regained in this phase if we refocus our efforts on finding the cause of what initially brought us to the path of imbalance. If that is achieved, then we can regain a state of balance!

If left unresolved, this stage can lead to a variety of distressing and uncomfortable sensations. These could include physical pain, but not always - sometimes we may feel no obvious symptoms at all. Still, if ignored for an extended period of time it will begin to take its toll on our bodies down the cellular level and spread into various tissues. The consequences are far-reaching: millions upon millions of cells in total are affected by these conditions when neglected!

If left without a reversal of the disease, it can spread to larger groups of tissues, which would then affect whole organs. It then moves onto whole systems and ultimately affects the entire being, resulting in the eventual death of the body. By lessening the effects of age-related illnesses, it is possible to extend your life and enjoy a higher quality of living. In this country, most deaths are no longer natural occurrences but instead can be attributed to degenerative processes.

Therefore, the key to overall health is found in correctly determining the relevant factors involved in health. This means managing health at a cellular level. Health is a consequence of choices one has made or hasn't made.

A Doctor's Approach to Health

Envision going to a doctor when you're in perfect health. Everything seems normal: your blood pressure, cholesterol, and weight are all within the recommended guidelines for someone of your age and height. If you tell them that what you desire is simply to remain this way, then they will likely exclaim "Fantastic!" Nevertheless, their advice might be nothing more than an encouragement to "carry on doing whatever it is that's working so well!"

The point is that this type of advice would only serve you for a limited amount of time. That is because the medical system is, at best, designed for early disease detection and symptom management, but not for prevention.

How would you react to a mechanic telling you that all you need to do for your car is to bring it in and have the oil changed when it starts to give you problems? We all know what that would do; we know what the consequences of not getting an oil change in time are for our car, which we only have for about ten years at best. Yet, we don't always give our bodies — which we will hopefully have for many decades — the same kind of preventative care.

Antibiotics & Dis-Ease

Why do we put so little effort into maintaining our bodies? That is due to the fact that most people believe in a magic pill that can solve all of their problems. However, no medicine has ever cured anyone; the body does the healing, and it happens no other way.

The birth of medicine could be attributed to the time when Robert Koch postulated the germ theory in 1860. Once this discovery occurred, it was emphasized and widely believed that microbes were the cause of disease. It was also widely accepted that the key to health lay in removing these microbian elements from the environment. This theory has however resulted in the overuse of antibiotics, leading to super-strains of bacteria and viruses. These microbes are now becoming increasingly resistant to all antibiotics that were created to fight them off!

Alternative Health Options

Today, people are beginning to realize that there is more than one path to good health. People are fed up with the status quo and want answers; they don't just want a generic diagnosis, or a medication prescribed without an explanation of why it will help them feel better. With this newfound awareness of alternative healthcare options, individuals can now make educated decisions about their well-being and be empowered through taking control of their own lives.

Our collective knowledge and understanding of health are improving. In 2001, the United States saw a vast increase in visits to alternative healthcare professionals instead of traditional allopathic medical doctors. This phenomenon was likely spurred by baby boomers who sought to better their physical condition without resorting to either medications or surgeries as a means for treatment. We are not helpless targets of the flu; rather, we create an ideal atmosphere that encourages microbial growth. Our body is teeming with toxins and other impurities, making it a veritable buffet for bacteria and viruses. Therefore, if we want to protect ourselves from infection caused by these microorganisms, then we must combat our toxic environment first!

To experience different results, switch up your mind frame! Everyone has the capability to alter their attitude and approach towards health. If you keep viewing your physical state in the same fashion as before little transformation will occur. So, if it's improvements you want to observe, begin by shifting your thought process today! It is essential to prioritize your health as something that should be actively maintained and even improved, not merely tolerated. In life, we regularly engage in the activities that are a priority for us; make sure you consider your well-being so noticeably important it becomes an unavoidable top concern.

To make your health a priority, you must realize that there are various choices we make every day that can be categorized into two broad areas: doing things that are important and urgent, and doing things that are important but not urgent.

To be the healthiest person you can be, devote your attention to matters which are truly meaningful and enriching - such as quality time with family, spiritual worship, workouts, proper nutrition, and intimate moments with a partner. These activities might not seem urgent, but they provide immense fulfilment! Remember that cultivating good health requires a consistent focus on what's important for you.

The key to achieving wellness is asking yourself, "What can I do today that will help me on my journey?" Small changes are often the easiest way to start. For instance, one of my patients hadn't worked out in years and was worried about getting back into it. But when she started by just stretching for 5 minutes a day, it quickly became 10 then 15 and eventually more! By taking those initial small steps you can ultimately achieve your goals. Subsequently, she felt incredibly invigorated while stretching and decided to incorporate some light resistance with weights in her routine. By the end of the month, not only had she added cardiovascular exercises but was exercising for half an hour daily! She found it so rewarding that making exercise part of her daily habits was now one of her top priorities.

After you form a habit, it's easy to take your progress even further. However, if you start with too much ambition, then chances are that things won't go as planned. What I would like for everyone to gain from this chapter is an understanding of how small decisions we make daily can have huge impacts on our overall health and well-being. The choices we make throughout the day play pivotal roles in deciding whether we stay healthy!

If you want to test out this theory, I have an assignment for you. First, get yourself a health journal; it can be any small notebook that you can keep with you. Next, write down the following on the inside cover or first page of your journal:

"At this moment, I hereby permit myself to bring my health to the highest level I was meant to experience by nurturing, taking care of, and forgiving myself as I would a loved one. I declare this today — a day that I will never forget — as the day my life and health were changed forever."

Your health journal should begin with a list of goals, which can be categorized into physical, mental, and spiritual. You may want to eat better; thus, be specific and list the types of foods you want to avoid, to obtain better health. If you plan on learning a new skill or improving a relationship, record specific actions that you can take over which you have complete control. The more specific you are, the more successful you will be.

Each day, record the small steps you have taken in your journal or notebook. Also, record your setbacks and shortcomings, as they will help you to see your progress over time.

How Can Chiropractic Care Affect Your Health?

The most significant way in which chiropractic can help you is by focusing not on your symptoms, but on the body's ability to regain a healthy state. You will never truly recover your body's health potential if you constantly chase symptoms. You will always be days or months away from your next appointment and should focus solely on relieving symptoms as quickly as possible! Chiropractic care allows you to shift your perception of going to the doctor only when there is a problem, to going to the chiropractor to maintain health.

Where would we be if we had a health care system where the doctors were only paid a salary, based on how healthy their patients are? Sound crazy? That's precisely what took place in ancient China: Doctors got paid based on how healthy their patients were. It does not impress me whatsoever when a doctor says, "It's a good thing you came in; we found some significant problems with you and need to go in for an immediate bypass or something equally invasive." Issues like that don't just appear out of nowhere; it takes years and years for such conditions to develop. Again, technology in the medical community heavily emphasizes early detection, rather than prevention.

Let's not solely point fingers at doctors here. Every one of us is accountable for our well-being, meaning that we must take preventative measures and make healthy choices to forestall the onset of illness. As parents, it is an absolute necessity to encourage our kids along a path towards lasting health through proper early care.

How Can Chiropractic Be A Strategy To Attain Good Health?

Any interference within or surrounding the nervous system causes disease or creates a situation where one is not entirely well. Often, this interference cannot be felt. There may be no pain or pressure to indicate something is not right. Sadly, it may take months or even years for symptoms to manifest themselves.

Research done by Professor Tzu claimed that pressure put on a nerve with the weight of only a dime can interfere with standard impulse transmissions, by up to 60%. It is staggering how little pressure it takes to reduce the body's ability to send corrective, healing messages out to all its vital systems. Chiropractic isn't about waiting until an issue arises and then swooping in to address the symptom, but not tackling its origin. Rather, it's focused on protecting your wellness and helping you stay at a higher level of functioning neurologically so that you can maintain optimal well-being without any underlying issues.

Visualize how your life would benefit if you applied this same rationale to every aspect. What gains could you make with your finances? How much stronger would relationships be — especially the most important one, with your spouse — if this preventative model was used all around? The results are clear; applying it in all areas will lead to a marked improvement in every part of your life. By proactively managing your health, you can avoid unnecessary crises and save yourself from prolonged waiting. Rather than being on the defensive, take charge of your health now by making it a top priority. Don't wait until an urgent situation arises; be proactive instead!

How Chiropractic Can Change Your Life

To nourish health and well-being, I have formulated a mind-body approach called IE Technology - Information and Empowerment. You can achieve remarkable outcomes by combining information with personal empowerment. Beliefs play a significant role in the equation; it would help if you laid out a mental framework that aligns with your desired reality — in other words, trust in things that are expected to transpire.

Next, it is important to understand the importance of exercise; it is not an option and cannot be justified by stating that you already work hard at your job, chase the kids around the house, or work in the garden. While these activities are a great start for getting into motion, they do not constitute a real workout. You must have a cardiovascular exercise for your health; one that challenges and works your heart! Remember, your heart is a muscle that needs to pump blood through your entire body every day, for a very long time. It would help if you challenged it once in a while so that it can be as strong as possible.

One of the most vital components in maintaining a healthy body is ensuring proper breathing. All tissues require oxygen, as they will suffer if deprived of it. Oxygen provides nourishment to both lungs and all cells throughout the body. Additionally, drinking enough water daily is essential for sustaining life-long wellness. Flushing out toxins from the body is essential. It's important to remember that our bodies are composed of 75% water and not coffee, tea or soda; these beverages only give us a false sense of energy. Caffeine addicts may disagree with this fact, but there is no denying it - none of those drinks has any true or sustaining power.

If there is one thing everyone should understand, it's that greens are essential for health. Eating plenty of leafy green vegetables during the week is among the most profound decisions you can make to better your well-being. To comprehend why plants, play such an integral role in this regard, consider photosynthesis – a process by which plants turn light into energy when exposed to sunlight outdoors and thus impart us with sustenance through their consumption.

Eating raw vegetables is paramount for reaping the full health benefits of greens, as cooked food destroys many vital enzymes. These particular compounds are essential to preserving good health. Additionally, consuming antioxidants in your diet can help reduce and combat free radical damage associated with ageing. Hence, a healthy intake of both uncooked veggies and antioxidant-rich fruits is key to maintaining optimal well-being! Stress, injuries, and the ingestion of processed foods can lead to an accumulation of free radicals in our bodies. These particles have a detrimental effect on our well-being; they can damage cells at a cellular level which results in weakened immunity systems, leaving us open to infection and illness.

A healthy diet requires the addition of beneficial fats and oils. Our bodies need these to form cell membranes, which are composed of two layers, called phospholipid bilayers. Unfortunately, most people consume too much unhealthy fat in their diets - current research indicates that up to 90% of us do not get enough beneficial oil! That is staggering, considering the connection between low levels of essential oils in our diets and cardiovascular disease, and the resulting list of degenerative disorders.

CHAPTER 3

THE HEALTH MODEL VS. THE SICK MODEL

One important and positive way to know that healthcare is changing is that it's moving from a "sick care" model to a "well care" model. What does that mean? Well, in years past most healthcare was provided on a reactive basis. Meaning, when you got sick, you went to the doctor; this is the "sick care" model. Today, healthcare is moving toward a "well care" model, in which a primary care practitioner (PCP) works with a patient regularly.

The Health Model (also known as the wellness model) is a theory of caring for clients and patients, which brings the focus from being sick over to preventative care. In the wellness model, there is a strong emphasis on holistic care, which encourages clients to take part in healthy activities that create a stronger body and mind and can ward off illnesses instead of relying on the traditional health system to care for a sick body. Wellness is not just a set of practices that are incorporated at the doctor's office, but rather a lifestyle change. Wellness includes care from your regular physician, but it can also include chiropractic, massage, nutrition, fitness, and mental health care. All of these things make you a healthier person.

Health Care vs. Sick Care

Health care is all about maintaining a healthy lifestyle. This can be achieved through various activities such as nutrition, exercise, dietary supplements, dental visits, chiropractic treatments and massage therapy - to name a few! Think of it like this: imagine there's an invisible spectrum with health at one end and illness at the other. Depending on your actions or behaviors you may move closer towards either side of the spectrum; so, if you want to stay in good health make sure that you take steps to "shift" back into healthier habits when necessary! When it comes to health, having a proactive attitude is key for the prevention of disease and promoting overall wellness. Taking action before any issues arise should be the primary focus. On the other hand, when sickness strikes or an illness is already present, then being reactive in order to address those medical crises becomes paramount.

Sick care is simply a defense measure. When it comes to emergency situations such as traumas and accidents, sick care becomes especially essential in order to avoid fatalities or permanent damage. Besides taking charge of acute conditions, the same model is implemented on chronic issues like diabetes, cancer and heart disease too; its key element being preventing further deterioration instead of finding what caused the problem initially. While making you feel better plays an important role here as well, restoring your health isn't something this system generally focuses on either - nor does it prevent similar problems from arising again in future.

The Wellness Approach

Wellness care seeks to turn on the natural healing ability, not by adding something to the system, but by removing anything which might interfere with normal functions, trusting that the body would know what to do if nothing was interfering with it. Standard medical care, on the other hand, seeks to treat a symptom by adding something from the outside - a medication, surgery or a certain procedure.

Wellness is a state of optimal conditions, for normal function and, it is an approach that looks for underlying causes of any disturbance or disruption, and take interventions and lifestyle adjustments which would optimize the conditions. That environment encourages natural healing and minimizes the need for invasive treatment, which should be administered only when necessary. When the body is working properly it tends to heal itself effectively, almost no matter what the condition is. When the body heals and maintains itself well, then there is another level of health which goes beyond "asymptomatic", or "pain-free", that reveals an opportunity for vitality, vibrant health and an enhanced experience of life. This is true for mental and emotional health, as well as physical health.

The Concepts Of Illness Behavior And Sick-Role Behavior In Healthcare

Generally, the behavior of healthy people and those who try to maintain their health are considered behaviors connected to the prevention of disease.

Such behaviors are intended to reduce susceptibility to disease, as well as reduce the effects of any diseases when they occur. The secondary prevention of disease is more closely related to the control of a disease, that an individual has, or which is incipient in the individual. Tertiary prevention is generally seen as directed toward reducing the impact and progression of symptomatic disease in an individual. This type of prediction is closely related to the concept of sick-role behavior.

The research from these principles of behavior has significantly aided in defining critical approaches to public health, in modern public health practice which is centered on community-based approaches, with an emphasis on participation

Now, researchers have a significant body of knowledge demonstrating the wide diversity in these behaviors regarding all the important demographic variables.

Research has been done which shows that the outcome of presenting symptoms to a physician is highly dependent on gender, ethnic background and other sociocultural characteristics. Research on the sick-role concept has elucidated the issue of power and its many manifestations in doctors' offices, hospitals, and other medical settings. This seems to indicate the serious role that power, and authority play in patient-physician interactions.

In general, illness and sick-role behaviors are viewed as characteristics of individuals and as concepts derived from sociological and socio-psychological theories.

Illness Behavior

The concept of illness behavior was used extensively throughout the second half of the twentieth century. Broadly speaking, it is any behavior undertaken by an individual who is ill, to relieve that experience or to better define the meaning of the disease experience. There are many different types of illness behavior that have been studied. Some individuals who experience physical or mental symptoms turn to the medical care system for help; others may turn to self-help strategies while others may decide to dismiss the symptoms. Illness behavior may be a mixture of behavioral decisions, too. For example, an individual faced with recurring symptoms of joint pain may turn to complementary or alternative medicine for relief. However, sudden sharp, debilitating symptoms may lead one directly to the hospital emergency room. In any event, illness behavior is usually mediated by strong subjective interpretations of the meaning of those symptoms. As with any type of human behavior, many social and psychological factors intervene and determine the type of illness behavior expressed in the individual.

The Health Belief Model

The Health Belief Model was developed by social scientists at the U.S. Public Health Service, to understand the failure of people in adopting disease prevention strategies or screening tests. The HBM suggests that a person's belief in the personal threat of an illness or disease, together with their belief in any effectiveness of the recommended health behavior, predicts the likelihood of how well that person adapts to the behavior. The Health Belief Model is a motivational framework that uses the desire to avoid a negative health consequence, as the prime motivation for taking positive health actions. HIV, for example, is a negative health consequence that people are motivated to avoid. This desire can be used to encourage sexually active people to practice safe sex. Similarly, the perceived threat of a heart attack can be used to motivate a person with high blood pressure into exercising more often. A negative health consequence is one of the key elements of the HBM.

The HBM derives from psychological and behavioral theory, with the foundation that the two components of health-related behavior are the desire to avoid illness, or conversely get well if already ill, and the belief that a specific health action will prevent or cure illness. Ultimately, an individual's course of action often depends on the person's perceptions of the benefits and barriers related to health behavior. There are six constructs of the HBM.

Perceived Susceptibility: This refers to a person's subjective perception of the risk of acquiring an illness or disease. There is wide variation in a person's feelings of personal vulnerability to an illness or disease.

Perceived Severity: This refers to a person's feelings on the seriousness of contracting an illness or disease (or leaving the illness or disease untreated). There is wide variation in a person's feelings of severity, and often a person considers the medical consequences (e.g., death, disability) and social consequences (e.g., family life, social relationships) when evaluating the severity.

Perceived Benefits: This refers to a person's perception of the effectiveness of various actions available to reduce the threat of illness or disease (or to cure illness or disease). When taking action to prevent or cure a disease, consideration, and evaluation of both perceived susceptibility and perceived benefit is required, as well as the willingness to accept the recommended health action if it is perceived as beneficial.

Perceived Barriers: This refers to a person's feelings on the obstacles to performing a recommended health action. There is wide variation in a person's feelings of barriers or impediments, which lead to a cost/benefit analysis. The person weighs the effectiveness of the actions against the perceptions that it may be expensive, dangerous (e.g., side effects), unpleasant (e.g., painful), time-consuming, or inconvenient.

Cue To Action: This is the stimulus needed to trigger the decision-making process to accept a recommended health action. These cues can be internal (e.g., chest pains, wheezing, etc.) or external (e.g., advice from others, illness of family member, newspaper article, etc.).

Self-Efficacy: This refers to the level of a person's confidence in his or her ability to successfully perform a behavior. This construct was added to the model most recently in mid-1980. Self-efficacy is a construct in many behavioral theories as it directly relates to whether a person performs the desired behavior.

Limitations of Health Belief Model

There are several limitations of the HBM which limit its utility in public health. Limitations of the model include the following:

- It does not account for a person's attitudes, beliefs or other individual determinants that dictate a person's acceptance of a health behavior.
- It does not consider behaviors that are habitual and thus may inform the decision-making process to accept a recommended action (e.g., smoking).
- It does not take into account behaviors that are performed for non-health related reasons such as social acceptability.
- It does not account for environmental or economic factors that may prohibit or promote the recommended action.
- It assumes that everyone has access to equal amounts of information on the illness or disease.

- It assumes that cues to action are widely prevalent in encouraging people to act and that "health" actions are the main goal in the decision-making process.

The HBM is more descriptive than explanatory and does not suggest a strategy for changing health-related actions. Early studies in preventive health behaviors, showed that perceived susceptibility, benefits, and barriers were consistently associated with the desired health behavior and perceived severity less so. For the most effective use of the model, it should be integrated with other models that account for the environmental context and suggest strategies for change.

Preventative Healthcare

Health is a state of wholeness in which your body knows its ever-changing needs and responds to those, all on its own. I believe that chiropractic care is a long-term form of preventative healthcare that maintains your body's nervous system to keep you in good health for a lifetime.

True chiropractic care in a principled practice believes that bodily health exists when the body is in a state of wholeness; it understands its own constantly changing needs, and can respond to them on its own. Chiropractic care doesn't heal injuries; rather, it helps the body to engage its own incredible natural healing abilities through a long-term routine of preventative healthcare maintenance for the nervous system.

Preventative healthcare focuses on your entire nervous system: Your brain, spinal cord and every one of the millions of nerve connections throughout your body. It monitors your entire body and all its needs, to help control and coordinate the necessary responses that allow the body to learn, adapt and maintain its health and wellness.

Preventative Care Vs. Sick Care

The common healthcare model in the United States is the sick care model. It only looks at your body when you are sick and then decides how to best treat these symptoms.

The preventative healthcare model is completely natural and doesn't rely on chemicals, looking at the root cause of your underlying health issues. It is focused entirely on correcting spinal subluxations to allow your whole nervous system to communicate better and increase the body's overall healing abilities. This improves your ability to adapt to stress, and a variety of health conditions and helps to restore you to normal, healthy, and optimal function. Chiropractic care can restore your natural healing ability and provide increased vitality, energy, bodily functions, and overall health.

Hospitals and the Wellness Sham

Furthermore, while hospitals and health systems may preach wellness, few offer comprehensive services designed to improve your health and well-being. Rather, they pay lip-service to this essential component of health care – viewing wellness more as a marketing opportunity, than a true effort to do everything in their power to minimize unnecessary and costly utilization of their medical services.

There's no surprise here, since the dominant reimbursement mechanism, the fee for service, rewards the provision of medical services – not maximization of the health of a defined population. As a result, we pay a very dear price.

How to Move from Sickness to Wellness

For some of our clients, this can be a big challenge and the reality is that moving from a sick state of mind to a wellness state of mind, is incredibly personal. It is possible to shift from a sick-care system that doles out interventions to manage the burden of chronic illness, to a positive health system that is a system focused on wellness, which minimizes unnecessary utilization by focusing on population health. However, it would take tremendous willpower for numerous constituents to achieve such a powerful transformation.

The key to transitioning from one model to the other is time and support. When we meet a new client who can benefit from the wellness model, we address their immediate issues and then create a positive and encouraging atmosphere that they can feel comfortable expanding into. If they've come to see us for chiropractic care, we may encourage them to support that function with a visit to one of our massage therapists, or to a fitness class. Treating the whole body with kindness and mindfulness is often all it takes to move a client from being "sick" to being "well".

Far short of transformational change, there are nonetheless small seeds of hope in the form of new, evolving reimbursement and delivery models, such as ACOs and medical homes that stress population health management. For providers who have been burned in the past by assuming the risk for a defined population, there's little enthusiasm for doing so again.

Our Role in Changing the System

More than three decades ago, Jim Fries gave us one of the keys to healing American healthcare; a silver bullet. The question is whether we have the perseverance to change the healthcare paradigm, as well as accept the personal responsibility for our health, which is essential to success. Below are the roles for each of us to play:

Government:

There needs to be dramatically increased spending on proven prevention programs, that can be administered at a local, state or federal level. There should also be greater rewards under governmental reimbursement programs, for those providers who embrace risk and demonstrate their ability to reduce the morbidity of a defined population.

Consumers/Patients:

We have to understand what it means to be prudent stewards of our health and the health of our families. We must understand the role that lifestyle choices play, in determining our health and how we might combat risk factors that imperil our future. For many of us, we will need access to resources that will aid us on this journey – particularly if we are socio-economically challenged, and thus find lifestyle change all the more difficult. As has been well demonstrated, the social determinants of health play a profound role in wellness and well-being.

Providers:

Healthcare executives need to take the moral high ground and do the right things for the communities they serve. One place to begin is with the development of a strategic wellness plan illustrating how wellness initiatives can be integrated into the very fabric of your hospital or health system's care model. Once developed and implemented, you can then reasonably assert that you do everything possible to minimize unnecessary consumption of health care resources while maximizing the health and well-being of your patients.

Insurers/Payers:

There needs to be an overwhelming pressure to partner more fully with providers on the assumption of risk, for the health and well-being of a defined population, thus accelerating the demise of fee-for-service medicine and its replacement with a reimbursement mechanism, that rewards wellness.

Employers: There have to be broader adoption and implementation of wellness programs that incorporate proven mechanisms for elevating the health and well-being of an employed population. Such programs will likely involve potent incentives for lifestyle modification by those employees at risk.

Conclusion

It's time to put "health" back in healthcare. Physicians must join forces with other healthcare practitioners, whose focus is on building health and wellness, not just managing disease and illness. Drugs and surgeries target the main complaint and symptoms, but they fail to address the cause of the problems plaguing current-day society. No amount of medication will address the true cause of degenerative diseases if the dysfunction within the body is not identified and restored. The irony is that the majority of the top 10 causes of death in modern society are all connected to diet and lifestyle, such as heart disease, certain cancers, diabetes, and Alzheimer's – to name a few. If the medical community had continued to honor the health-building values of diet and exercise, these conditions would never have grown to their current proportions.

CHAPTER 4

THE GERM THEORY DEBUNKED

Germs are everywhere — in the food we eat, the air we breathe, the water we drink, and even inside our bodies. The term "germs" generally refers to microscopic organisms like bacteria, viruses, fungi, and protozoa. Minute as they are, germs are one of the most misunderstood aspects of health. The "germ theory" that most people use to explain disease with is a carry-over from the early 1800s. The theory states that specific germs can cause specific diseases, when our bodies provide a hospitable environment for them to reproduce in.

Germ theory denialism is the belief that germs do not cause infectious diseases, and that Pasteur's theory is inaccurate. This usually involves arguing that Louis Pasteur's model of infectious disease was incorrect and that Antoine Béchamp's was right. One of the first movements to deny the germ theory was the Sanitary Movement, which nonetheless was central in the development of America's public health infrastructure. One well-known advocate of this form of denialism is Bill Maher, who claimed that Pasteur recanted the germ theory on his deathbed. Several sources then began dubbing Maher as a "germ theory denialist", after his supposedly eccentric statements regarding Pasteur's theory.

In response to criticism of his views, Maher said, on the October 16, 2009, episode of his show, that he accepted microorganisms as the cause of some diseases. However, he expressed skepticism about other topics in medicine, such as vaccination. Similarly, the following month, Maher wrote that he "understand[s] germ theory" but he still thought that since the terrain in which bacteria can thrive is crucial and often controllable, it shouldn't even be controversial.

Who Was Louis Pasteur?

Louis Pasteur was born in Dole, Eastern France in 1822. He was a conscientious and hard-working student, though not considered exceptional. In fact, one of his own professors called him "mediocre." He received a doctorate in 1847 and after obtaining posts at Strasbourg, Lille, and Paris, he spent a long period researching various aspects of chemistry. Here, he studied tartaric acid - an acid found in wine - and discovered the existence of crystals that are mirror images of the compound.

His most important discoveries were in the field of germ study. He showed that germs required certain conditions to grow, and, using this knowledge, he found that the fermentation of yeast could be delayed. He also discovered practical ways of killing bacteria in organic liquids, such as milk. His process of heating milk to a high temperature and at a specific time successfully killed all the bacteria, without destroying the milk proteins. This was a radical discovery and made milk safer to drink. This process, known as pasteurization, was named after him and has since then saved many lives.

Louis Pasteur was a great believer in hard work, and never rested on his laurels. He continued to work in his laboratory to research further processes and cures for an array of conditions. In 1860, the French Academy announced a prize of 2,500 francs to anyone who could provide convincing experimental proof for or against the spontaneous generation of life.

Pasteur was awarded the prize in 1862 after he proved that no microbes ever grew in nutrient solutions which had been sterilized by heating, provided the air above the solutions was also sterilized. If unsterilized air was allowed into the space above the solutions, however, microbes would begin to grow in the solutions. He thereby proved that microbes are fount ever-present in our air and that sterilization can kill them.

The Pasteur Institute was opened in 1888. During Louis Pasteur's lifetime, it was not easy for him to convince others of his ideas — highly controversial in their time but considered absolutely correct today.

Pasteur fought to convince surgeons that germs existed and carried diseases, and that dirty hands and unsterilized medical instruments spread germs and, therefore, diseases. His pasteurization process killed germs and prevented the spread of disease.

Louis Pasteur had great faith in the goodness of humans. He worked tirelessly to provide real benefits for the treatment of infectious diseases. More than any other person, Louis Pasteur helped to increase average life expectancy in the late 19th and early 20th centuries.

Achievements of Louis Pasteur

- Process of pasteurization to make milk safe to drink.
- Cure for rabies
- Cure for anthrax
- His principles were used by later scientists such as Frankland, Valley Radot, Emile Duclaux, Descours and Holmes in developing vaccines for other diseases such as typhus, diphtheria, cholera, yellow fever, and different strains of plague.

How Did He Discover The Germ Theory?

Proving the germ theory of disease would later be known as the crowning achievement of Louis Pasteur. While he was not the first to propose the theory that diseases were caused by microscopic organisms, the view itself was controversial in the 19th century and opposed the previously accepted theory of "spontaneous generation."

Pasteur set out to understand the fermentation process. He soon realized that alcohol in wine was produced by yeasts that lived on the skins of grapes, and that during fermentation the yeast appeared healthy and budding under a microscope. However, when lactic acid was formed the wine turned to vinegar and other microbes were seen among the yeast cells. Further analysis of the wine showed a number of complex organic molecules, some of which were able to rotate light, a property of compounds produced by living organisms. Through several experiments, Pasteur showed that fermentation required contact with atmospheric dust from the air.

Pasteur then turned his attention to the health of silkworms, which produced silk for the cloth industry. He discovered that healthy silkworms became ill when they nested in the bedding of those that had suffered from silkworm nosema disease and flacherie. In this study, Pasteur found that the environment directly affected a contagion and that the spread of disease could be controlled by sterilization. His studies with yeasts had shown that microbes could be airborne, and he realized that these two studies could be directly applied to the transmission of diseases in humans.

The final proof of germ theory came about when Pasteur was able to grow anthrax bacilli in a culture. Although anthrax had been isolated by Robert Koch, opponents believed that the spores he found could have been contaminants in his culture medium. Pasteur placed a drop of blood from a sheep dying of anthrax into a sterile culture and allowed the bacilli to grow. He repeated this process until none of the original cultures remained in the final dish. The final culture produced anthrax when injected into sheep, showing that the organism was responsible for the disease.

Why Is The Germ Theory Considered Incorrect?

According to Louis Pasteur's widely accepted germ theory, many illnesses are carried by these microorganisms. Therefore, we must protect ourselves and our children from them. However, our body's entire ecosystem relies on symbiotic interactions with many bacteria, and our human digestion could not function properly without certain key bacteria that are essential for our digestive processes, such as Bacteroidetes and Firmicutes. So, what are they then? Are they friends or foes?

Let us revisit the germ theory: Suppose we are at the mercy of these little foes called bacteria and viruses found in our environment. In that case, why aren't we all affected and get ill? Have you ever wondered why a group of people exposed to an equal amount of the same germs respond differently? Take the recent swine flu as an example — why did some die, some get sick to then recover, while others yet remained unaffected? If we were truly only at the full mercy of this virus, wouldn't we all be dead by now? This may sound a little extreme, but why are some affected, and others left untouched? Is it bad luck? Is it simply chance? Or could there be other factors influencing the outcome here?

Germs are scientifically classified as opportunistic organisms. This means that they can only "attack" if - and only if - they are given the opportunity. This opportunity refers to a weak host or a person with a weakened immune system. If your immune system is weak, you have now become a target or an opportunity for a viral or bacterial attack. This can easily be observed in the increased susceptibility of the elderly, the very young, or in the case of people with extreme immunodeficiencies, such as those struggling with AIDS or some forms of cancer treatments that diminish the immune system. For example, for an AIDS patient, a common cold can be a fatal risk, due to the decreased functioning of their immune system. So, are germs really to blame? Are we victims of germs? Or are we victims of a weakened immune system? This is the main reason why this germ theory is considered incorrect by some.

Why Is The Terrain Or The Environment Considered To Be More Important Than The Germ?

The germ theory of disease is based on the concept that many diseases are caused by microorganisms, and although their growth and productive replication may be the cause of disease, environmental and genetic factors may predispose a host or influence the severity of the infection itself. For example, in a host that is immunocompromised (e.g., due to AIDS, old age, or other preexisting conditions), an infection may result in more severe outcomes than in fully immunocompetent individuals.

However, in 1876, Robert Koch was struggling to convince the world that germs cause disease. Today, environmental degradation is a pervasive planetary disease, but the causes remain shrouded in the same popular murk that made diseases mysterious before Koch and Louis Pasteur. For environmental issues, such as the decline of coral reefs, skeptics demand detailed evidence — we must know the exact cause and show that any proposed cures will work.

A commonly accepted story claims that Pasteur himself, in one of the most quoted deathbed statements of all time, recanted his own theory and admitted that his rival, Antoine Bechamp, had been right all along; that it was not the germ that caused disease, but rather the environment in which the germ was found (i.e., the "terrain").

What Is The Host Theory?

In the host theory, people don't "catch" germs which then give them diseases. Instead, disease-causing germs are actually opportunistic organisms that thrive in people whose bodies are weakened, or suffer an internal imbalance.

They are a byproduct of the disease, not a cause of the disease. You see, you have methicillin-resistant Staphylococcus aureus (MRSA), cancer, viruses, and bacteria in you and on you all the time, every day! A healthy balance of beneficial bacteria and a healthy environment of the body keeps all the unhealthy elements out and keeps the body in balance. However, suppose you wiped out everything using antibacterial soaps all the time, or by the use of antibiotics for every little cold you ever had. In that case, you wouldn't only be destroying the "bad bacteria", you would be effectively wiping out all bacteria - including the symbiosis you body has with beneficial bacteria, too, leaving you even more susceptible to further diseases and illness.

Unlike Pasteur, who spawned a mentality of fearful extermination of germs to prevent disease, Béchamp essentially understood the balance and importance of the internal environments we create with our food, so that our internal systems either protect us from or do not support disease.

Béchamp theorized that germs were actually the chemical byproducts and degenerative aspects of an unbalanced state of the body. For a disease to take hold, cellular dysfunction, damaged tissues, inflamed areas of the body, and other things had to be present. This is when germs or bacteria show up in excess — because the body, or an area of it, is in a state that allows them to thrive and reproduce unchecked. This cellular dysfunction or dead tissue can be caused by several things such as malnutrition or exposure to toxins.

As you can see, the host theory and germ theory are two radically different views of how people acquire the disease.

Who Was Antoine Béchamp?

Pierre Jacques Antoine Béchamp (October 16, 1816 – April 15, 1908) was a French scientist, now best known for his breakthroughs in applied organic chemistry and a bitter rivalry with Louis Pasteur. He was educated at the University of Strasbourg, receiving a Doctor of Science degree in 1853 and a Doctor of Medicine in 1856. Aside from that, he ran a pharmacy in the city. In 1854, he was appointed Professor of Chemistry at the University of Strasbourg — a post previously held by Louis Pasteur.

Béchamp developed the Béchamp reduction, an inexpensive method to produce aniline dye, permitting Perkin to launch the synthetic-dye industry. Béchamp also synthesized the first organic arsenical drug, arsanilic acid, from which Ehrlich later synthesized the first chemotherapeutic drug. Béchamp's rivalry with Pasteur was initially for priority in attributing fermentation to microorganisms. It was later for attributing the silkworm disease pebrine to microorganisms, and eventually over the validity of germ theory.

Béchamp also disputed cell theory. Claiming the discovery that the "molecular granulations" in biological fluids were actually the elementary units of life, Béchamp named them microzymas—that is, "tiny enzymes"—and credited them with producing both enzymes and cells while "evolving" amid favorable conditions into multicellular organisms. Denying that bacteria could invade a healthy animal and cause disease.

Bechamp claimed instead that unfavorable host and environmental conditions destabilize the host's native microzymas, after which they decompose host tissue by producing pathogenic bacteria. While both cell theory and germ theory gained widespread acceptance, granular theories became obscure. Bechamp's version, the microzymas theory, has been retained by small groups, especially in alternative medicine.

Why Was Rivalry Between Pasteur and Bechamp?

In 19th century France, while Pasteur was advocating the notion of germs as the cause of disease, Antoine Bechamp advocated a conflicting theory known as the "cellular theory" of disease.

Although Antoine Bechamp had his own incredible list of scientist appointments during his lifetime, he was overshadowed by Pasteur, the most celebrated scientist of the 19th century. Some call Bechamp the "Father of Modern Medicine," a title quite remarkable as Pasteur was not actually a physician. Nevertheless, both men were highly-regarded members of the French Academy of Science and submitted their scientific findings to the Academy for review and publication.

Because Bechamp frequently criticized Pasteur's work, an intense rivalry and feud between the two intensified in the Academy. But no matter how carefully Bechamp argued against some of Pasteur's scientific methods and conclusions, the Academy constantly gave approval to Pasteur.

Bechamp's cellular theory is almost completely opposite to that of Pasteur's: He noted that these germs that Pasteur was so terrified of were opportunistic in nature; they were everywhere and even existed inside of us in a symbiotic relationship. Bechamp noticed in his research that it was only when the tissue of the host became damaged or compromised, that these germs began to manifest as a prevailing symptom (not cause) of disease.

To prevent illness, Bechamp advocated not the killing of germs but the cultivation of health through diet, hygiene, and healthy lifestyle practices like exercise. The idea is that if a person has a strong immune system and good tissue quality (or "terrain" as Bechamp called it), the germs will not manifest in the person, and he/she will have good health. It is only when their health starts to decline (due to personal neglect and poor lifestyle choices) that they become susceptible to infections.

You can see this when a group of people goes hiking in the woods. It often seems that the mosquitoes attack only one or two people out of the group. As it turns out, it's always the same person who is constantly attacked by mosquitoes. This person is also often the one who always catches the latest flu and has the weakest immune system. This is because these germs (including insects) are opportunistic in nature and only attack the weak.

Bechamp's cellular theory also applies in treating illnesses. Bechamp was less concerned with killing the illness and focused more on restoring the health of the patient's body through healthy lifestyle choices. Bechamp saw infection as a footnote to the state of illness and not as the primary cause. As the person's health is restored through diet, hygiene, and detoxification, the infection went away on its own without needing measures to kill it.

Pasteur and Bechamp had a long and often bitter rivalry regarding who was right about the actual cause of illness. Ultimately, Pasteur's ideas were more widely accepted by society, and Bechamp was pretty much forgotten in history. The practice of Western medicine is today mainly based on Pasteur's germ phobia, which gives rise to the use of vaccinations, antibiotics, and other antimicrobials.

The irony is that towards the end of his life, Pasteur seems to have renounced the germ theory altogether and admitted that Bechamp was right all along. In the 1920s, medical historians also discovered that most of Pasteur's theories turned out to be plagiarized from Bechamp's early research work.

What Is The Real Truth Behind The Human Body Around Germs?

The human genome is made up of about 23,000 genes. That's a reasonably impressive figure, until you consider this: the number of non-human genes each of us carry around, from the bacteria, viruses and other pathogens living in and on us, totals eight million. Most of the cells in the human body also aren't even human in nature! Indeed, bacterial cells easily outnumber human cells if a 10 - 1 ratio. This is why the exploration of the human microbiome, the collective population of all the non-human cells and genes which inhabit us, has become one of the fastest-rising fields of medical research.

What scientists are discovering is that these microbes are not just freeloaders or invaders; rather, they are crucial facilitators of many of our basic bodily functions, from digesting food and producing vitamins, to fending off harmful infections and helping us recover from illness. They not only keep us healthy, but they may also explain differences in individual health - the reason why people respond differently to the same drug, or why some people develop chronic diseases and others don't.

Food, water, and even the air can be made dangerous to living organisms if they are exposed to something harmful. When this happens, that element is said to be contaminated, toxic or polluted.

Harmful germs can easily enter the body through the mouth, nose, eyes, and genitals (privates), and even enter through the skin itself. Once disease-causing germs are inside the body, they may grow very quickly under the perfect conditions — a small number of germs can easily become millions in no time. As an example, a study with obese subjects showed a dominating presence of Firmicutes (a group of bacteria that produce butyrate, a substance which helps keep our colon healthy) to Bacteroidetes (another group of bacteria, which help support the microbiome of our gut), and that obese patients had a much larger bacterial diversity in their intestines. Furthermore, another study showed that a predominance of Firmicutes to Bacteroidetes can lead to more fat accumulation and obesity.

Our guts are home to a vast array of beneficial bacteria, essential for good health and functioning. These bacteria, known as probiotics, help to support digestion and the absorption of nutrients from food, prevent harmful bacteria from invading our bodies and producing toxins, boost our immune systems, reduce inflammation and even play a role in producing vitamins. It is becoming increasingly clear that the human microbiome plays an integral role in maintaining our health. It is important to remember that it is not just what we eat, but also how we are exposed to bacteria and other microorganisms, that determines our overall health.

CHAPTER 5

THE IMPORTANCE OF EPIGENETICS

Epigenetics is a field of study that investigates external changes to genes that can be inherited, but do not involve changes to the DNA sequence. Such changes may be caused by age, diet, exercise, relationships, sleep, emotions, stress, mindset, environment, lifestyle choices and diseases. These phenotypic changes without a corresponding genotypical change can cause misreading of the genes in cells, leading to disorders in organs and even severe diseases such as cancer.

Epigenetics holds the secret of how diseases develop and how early aging occurs. We can no longer blame our genes for everything, as a lot of what happens to our bodies is caused by our choices and environment. Also, we cannot just change our diet, start exercising, and be satisfied that we will be healthy; there is more to health, and much of it lies in the cells.

Telomeres

The human body comprises bones, muscles, glands, organs, and much else. Each of these is made up of specific types of cells, and each cell has certain components, with the nucleus located at the center. The nucleus contains structures called chromosomes; these are actually "packages" of DNA arranged into chromosomes that contain all the genetic information passed down from parents to their children. The chromosomes come in pairs, forming our cellular alphabet and providing the instructions needed to construct our bodies. In order for growth to occur, our bodies duplicate their cells through cell division, or mitosis. During mitosis, one "parent" cell divides into two new "daughter" cells. During this process, cells make copies of their genetic material so that each daughter cell contains the same information as the original cell.

Each DNA strand is protected at each end by telomeres, DNA sequences, and proteins, ensuring that the information is passed on from one generation to the next. Telomeres protect chromosomes from damage and fusion with neighboring chromosomes, similar to how shoelace caps protect shoelaces from fraying. Telomeres are essential; without them, DNA strands become damaged, resulting in malfunctioning cells.

Telomeres shorten naturally and gradually each time a cell divides, thus leading to the body's gradual aging. Once they shorten to a certain length, the cells stop dividing and die. However, evidence suggests that damage to telomeres can make them shrink faster than usual. Damage to telomeres causes damage to the DNA, resulting in poor cell health, which leads to early aging and disease.

Factors Negatively Affecting Telomeres

Many factors affect telomeres, causing acceleration of the rate at which they shorten.

1. <u>Diet</u> is the most potent factor that can damage telomeres, considering that we eat and drink several times a day; we damage body cells when we consume the following:

- Animals in industrial farm settings are fed products that contain growth hormones, antibiotics, and other chemicals.
- Processed foods contain synthetic flavors, preservatives, colorants, taste enhancers, and many other potentially harmful chemicals.
- Too much sugar can make the body acidic and impair the pancreas.
- Artificial sweeteners harm the brain and nerves.
- Intensively farmed fruits, vegetables, and grains are sprayed with harmful pesticides and herbicides.
- Fish, full of pollutants (including mercury), are allowed into our rivers and oceans.

2. <u>Water</u> treated with fluoride is known to be harmful and carcinogenic. We absorb fluoride when we drink, bathe, or shower in this type of water.

3. <u>Medicines</u> used in conventional medical practices can be harmful due to inorganic chemicals that shorten telomerase. They work by suppressing specific natural body processes. Read any leaflet enclosed with your medicine, and you will see a list of side effects. The longer one takes a particular drug, the greater the risk of developing health problems that were not present beforehand. That is why people on chronic medication often have an extensive list of illnesses.

4. <u>Personal care products</u> often contain a lengthy list of potentially harmful chemicals. By the time you finish shaving, bathing, shampooing, cleansing your face, moisturizing and applying makeup, you have put dozens of toxic substances onto your body; these may include parabens, synthetic colors, synthetic fragrances, sodium lauryl sulfate, formaldehyde, 1,4 dioxane, phthalates, polyethylene glycol (PEGs), petroleum jelly (petrolatum), mineral oil, BHA (butylated hydroxyanisole), BHT (butylated hydroxytoluene), retinyl palmitate, triethanolamine (TEA), triclosan, DEA (diethanolamine), cocamide DEA and lauramide DEA.

The list is endless; each item one applies to their body has a specific effect that they want, but this is often made possible due to harmful chemicals. Searching the internet for each of these ingredients will shock one by how much they affect our health.

5. <u>Laundry and cleaning products</u>, such as air fresheners, drain cleaners, detergents, bleaches, fabric softeners, scourers, polishes and cleaners that we use in our home, all contain inorganic chemicals which can harm cells and

affect our health in many ways. We absorb these chemicals through ingestion, inhalation, or absorption through the skin. Some harmful ingredients are phthalates, triclosan, quaternary ammonium compounds (or "Quats"), ammonia, chlorine, sodium hydroxide, 2-butoxyethanol, synthetic colors, synthetic fragrances, and many others.

If they advertise a product's new, better cleaning qualities, know that yet another harmful ingredient has probably been added. Search the internet for some of these ingredients and see how they can harm our health.

6. Cigarettes. Researchers have found a strong association between smoking and accelerated shortening of telomeres, which accelerates aging. A person who smokes one pack of cigarettes per day for 40 years can accelerate their aging by 7.4 years due to the hundreds of chemicals present in tar, a component of cigarettes, which can poison body cells.

7. Stress is another unsuspected factor that harms our telomeres. Money problems, long working hours, heavy workloads, and caregiving for family members have made life highly stressful for many. Research has found a strong link between chronic psychological stress and the accelerated shortening of telomeres. Stress is one of the most important factors responsible for telomere shortening.

8. Obesity has also been linked to rapid telomere shortening. Obesity causes increased oxidative stress, which induces DNA damage and a shortening of the telomeres. The research found that the telomeres in obese

women were significantly shorter than those in lean women of the same age group.

Researchers have calculated that the excessive loss of telomeres in obese individuals is equivalent to 8.8 years of life, an effect that is possibly worse than smoking. All in all, these findings indicate that obesity negatively affects telomeres and may even accelerate the aging process.

9. Caffeine shortens telomeres, according to Professor Martin Kupiec of Tel Aviv University and his colleagues. They expanded on a 2004 study by Nobel Prize-winning molecular biologist Professor Elizabeth Blackburn, which discovered that emotional stress shortens telomeres, presumably by generating free radicals in the cells.

In their study, Professor Martin Kupiec and his colleagues grew yeast cells in conditions that generated free radicals to test the effect on telomere length. Then, they exposed the yeast cells to various environmental stressors. When they were exposed to a low concentration of caffeine, similar to the levels found in a shot of espresso, the telomeres were shortened. Thus, it can be concluded that caffeine shortens telomeres and is detrimental to one's health.

11. Alcohol. A study on 200 known abusers of alcohol was conducted to investigate the effect of alcohol abuse on telomere length in peripheral blood leukocytes. The control group consisted of 257 social drinkers. It was found that the telomere length in alcohol abusers was

almost halved compared to the telomere length in the control group.

It was also found that telomere length decreased with increased units of drink per day. Those who drank more than four units per day had substantially shorter telomere lengths than those who drank fewer than four units per day.

12. <u>Environmental pollution</u> also affects telomere length. Researchers evaluated telomere length in the leukocytes taken from office workers and traffic police officers exposed to traffic pollution. The levels of toluene and benzene indicated exposure to pollution. The researchers found that, for each age group, the telomere length in the traffic police officers was shorter than that of the office workers. This is clear proof that pollution affects health by shortening telomeres.

In another research, the lymphocytes of coke-oven workers exposed to polycyclic aromatic hydrocarbons were found to have significantly shorter telomeres, increased evidence of DNA damage, and genetic instability compared to control subjects. Moreover, a reduction in telomere length in these workers was significantly linked to the number of years they were exposed to the chemicals. It is well known that coke-oven workers are at a high risk of developing lung cancer, and that telomere shortening has been associated with an increased risk of cancer development and early aging.

Working in polluted environments can increase the risk of cancer and other diseases, as well as accelerate the rate of aging by shortening telomeres.

Factors Positively Affecting Telomeres

1. <u>Moderate alcohol consumption</u> lengthens telomeres, as Professor Martin Kupiec and his colleagues have found. This explains why moderate drinking reduces the risks of cancer, heart disease, and strokes.

2. <u>Dietary fiber</u> was found to be positively linked to telomere lengthening, implying that it is healthier to eat a fiber-rich diet.

3. <u>A reduction in protein</u> intake has been found to positively affect telomere length and increase longevity. In a study involving rats, a 40% reduction of protein led to a 15% increase in the lifespan of the rodents. The rats were subjected to a protein-restricted diet early in life, after which they showed a long-term suppression of appetite, a reduced growth rate, and an increased lifespan. It was found that the increased lifespan in the animals was associated with significantly longer telomeres in their kidneys.

This may explain why Japanese people have the highest life expectancy, which is associated with a low-protein intake and a high-carbohydrate diet. The source of protein is also an essential factor; for example, replacing casein with soy protein in rats was associated with a delayed incidence of chronic kidney disease and an increased lifespan.

4. <u>Antioxidants</u> reduce the shortening of telomeres. Farzaneh-Far and others studied the relationship between omega-3 fatty acid levels in the blood and

temporal changes in telomere length. The study involved 608 heart disease patients who were recruited from the Heart and Soul Study between September 2000 and December 2002. The researchers followed omega-3 fatty acid levels and telomere length in these individuals until January 2009.

They found that a diet containing antioxidant omega-3 fatty acids reduced the rate of telomere shortening. They also found that a lack of these antioxidants was associated with an increased rate of telomere shortening. This proved that antioxidants reduce the rate of telomere shortening.

Another study found that women who consumed an antioxidant with a poor diet were at a moderate risk of developing breast cancer and had shorter telomeres. It was also discovered that a diet rich in antioxidants, such as vitamin E, vitamin C, and beta-carotene, led to longer telomeres and a lower risk of developing breast cancer. Therefore, it can be concluded that a diet rich in antioxidants can help protect telomeres from damage.

5. <u>Dietary restrictions</u> have been passed down for millennia, and periodic fasting is recommended as a way to preserve telomere length. Finally, scientific research has proven this to be true. In a study involving animals, restricting food intake slowed growth and promoted longer life. The explanation for this phenomenon is that reduced food intake reduces the oxidative burden on the cells, which reduces DNA damage and therefore keeps animals biologically younger for longer periods of time.

6. <u>Exercising</u> reduces telomere shortening; it is suspected that this reduction of telomeres is due to exercise reducing oxidative stress and elevating the expression of proteins that stabilize telomeres, potentially slowing aging and age-associated diseases. This can be achieved by increasing the elimination of toxins from the body and decreasing the amount of fat in one's body.

Telomerase

Telomerase is an enzyme that prevents the rapid shortening of telomeres, leading to cell death. This enzyme is also known as telomere terminal transferase (TTT). It is highly active in fetal and adult stem cells, but it shows a decline in activity in normal cells as we grow older. Interestingly, telomerase is very active in cancer cells.

Understanding telomerase is crucial, as it is the key to longevity. There is convincing evidence that the length of a person's life is dictated by the limited number of times a human cell can divide. The clock starts ticking when the reproductive cell transforms into a developmental cell in the developing embryo, and the cell's fate is predestined to a limited 75 to 100 cell divisions. The length of the telomeres goes down by 100 bases per cell division; by the time of birth, the size of the telomeres has already shrunk from 15,000 base pairs to 10,000 base pairs. The length of the telomeres continues to shrink until it reaches 5,000 base pairs, at which point the cell cannot divide anymore. These cells are then biologically "old," and a body eventually starts to decay or deteriorate due to diseases.

However, telomerase plays a crucial role in regulating the lifespan of cell production. Telomerase activity is very much involved in and necessary for cell development, aging, and transforming normal cells into cancer cells. The implication is that if we can improve telomerase activity, we can prevent or slow down the shortening of telomeres. As a result, cells can continue to grow and divide normally. If we can do this, we can prevent aging; in other words, we can reset our biological clock!

Factors Affecting the Activation of Telomerase

Telomerase activation is needed for the self-renewal and production of several cell types, including cancer cells, activated lymphocytes, and stem cells. Under laboratory conditions, introducing telomerase into cultured human cells alters the aging of human cells into immortal cells without transforming them into cancer cells. Cells with shortened telomeres can remain genetically stable if the enzyme telomerase is operational; therefore, it is important to know what affects telomerase activation and make lifestyle changes accordingly.

1. Exercise has been shown to elevate telomerase activity in mice, according to research. Studies involving humans have found that leukocytes derived from athletes had increased telomerase activity and reduced telomere shortening, compared to those of non-athletes.

2. Calorie restriction increases telomerase activity, as found in a study involving laboratory rats.

3. <u>Meditation</u> increases telomerase activity, as found in an 8-week study that involved caregivers for patients with dementia.

4. <u>Improvements in nutrition</u> and lifestyle have been shown to increase telomerase activity, as was proven by Dr. Dean Ornish's study involving 30 men with low-risk prostate cancer. He changed their diet to a "low-fat" (10% of calories from fat), whole foods, plant-based diet that centered on vegetables, fruits, unrefined grains, and legumes; intake of refined carbohydrates was minimized.

The diet was supplemented with soy (one daily serving of tofu, plus 58 g of a fortified soy protein powder beverage), fish oil (3 g per day), vitamin E (100 IU per day), selenium (200 µg per day), and vitamin C (2 g per day). The subjects also had moderate aerobic exercise (walking 30 minutes per day, six days per week); stress management (meditation, gentle yoga-based stretching, imagery, breathing, and progressive relaxation techniques 60 minutes per day, six days per week), and a one-hour group support session once per week. Participants also met with staff members for four hours per week and had one weekly telephone contact with a study nurse.

After three months, researchers found that there was increased telomerase activity accompanied by decreases in perceived psychological distress and LDL cholesterol.

5. <u>Vitamin D</u> increases telomerase activity, as was found in a study.

How Chiropractic Care Affects Our Epigenetic Expression

When a person suffers from subluxation (partial dislocation of a joint), several physiological and biomechanical problems can develop, such as hyperemia, edema, congestion, minute hemorrhages, scarring, ischemia (muscle pain), muscle atrophy, and tissue rigidity. Subluxation can seriously affect the quality of life by distorting an individual's perception of the environment and compromising their ability to respond to it.

Therefore, when a chiropractor adjusts, they make a considerable change that goes deeper than just the physical. After the adjustment, patients usually report a heightened state of well-being and perceptual awareness. By simply manipulating a specific part of the body, the chiropractor may have been affecting the patient's genetic expression and the bodies and brains of the patient's descendants.

Correction of vertebral subluxation may affect genetic mechanisms in two ways:

— The chiropractor might have an impact on basic physiological processes that affect DNA repair and oxidative stress.
— The patient's perception of the environment may change, and constructive and appropriate responses to the environment may develop, completely changing the patient's life.

The chiropractor is in a perfect position to facilitate the determination of humanity's legacy. That is a lot of power!

CHAPTER 6

WELLNESS AND PREVENTION

Prevention is better than cure. If you can keep yourself healthy through diet, exercise, and controlling stress, you are much better off than dealing with diseases or conditions which are a product of poor lifestyle choices.

Choosing to live a healthy lifestyle and care not only for your spine but also for every part of the body and mind, should be a simple choice. No one wants to be unhealthy. No one wants pain. No one wants to be limited in their movement or abilities, either physical or mental.

Sometimes it is only a matter of knowing what to do and how to do it. You want results, but you are still trying to figure out how to get from point A to point B. This is where I come in. As a chiropractor, personally and professionally, I have committed myself to educating others on how to get the most out of their body and, in turn, get the most out of living a healthy, pain-free, and illness-free life.

Now, I am not saying that if you consistently eat right, exercise, lift safely and move properly, you will never get sick or injured. All I am stating is that you will have increased the likelihood of your body being prepared to handle the external forces placed upon it. With good nutrition and exercise, for example, you are naturally creating a more robust immune system against toxins found in the air, along with viruses brought on and spread by others. You are creating a solid, natural defense against a myriad of diseases.

Exercise and good diet help to build strong bones and muscles. An impact-related injury then is less likely to occur, and the body is better protected against accidents. A spine kept in alignment, through preventative chiropractic care, is more easily corrected through a minor adjustment, following an injury. Again, you are keeping the spine free from blockage or subluxation that can prevent the body from repairing what may be wrong and keeping itself healthy. Yes, the saying that an ounce of prevention is worth a ton of cure has never been truer than when it comes to your health and well-being.

Managing Stress

Far too little emphasis is placed on the reality that emotional stress, mental trauma, and phobias can cause real, damaging physical reactions and responses in the body. When you are emotionally stressed, subtle changes take place in your posture, which puts strain on the joints and muscles. This in turn leaves them susceptible to injury. Severe mental stress can even cause actual compression of spinal joints.

There are many successful ways to reduce stress. One method may work perfectly for one person, while another may need to try a different approach. Managing stress is a highly individual process. No two people can go about it the same way. The key here is to find out what works best for you and to apply it whenever necessary.

There are some basic categories for reducing stress. Within one of these, you will probably find a more specific method that works for you. The goal is to control the mind's stress levels, with a mental or physical activity that brings about material changes, such as slowing the heart rate, lowering blood pressure and releasing muscle tension, etc. Any physical change brought about by mental stress, such as deadlines, pressure at work, or financial worries, can also be reverted to a more desirable state, through stress-reduction techniques.

Stress-Reducing Exercises

Exercise has so many benefits, one of which is reducing stress. In practice, this can entail a shorter visit to the local gym, changing into specific clothing, and formally doing calisthenics, but exercise is simply moving the body to get the heart pumping, and blood flowing, so that endorphins can be released. Endorphins are hormonal chemicals that give you a feeling of elation and are connected to physical and mental wellness. Some people even refer to it as a natural "high".

Here are some great exercises requiring no equipment, except good shoes and very little preparation. They can be done at a moment's notice, which helps reduce stress and refreshes the mind and body.

- Take a brisk 20-minute walk in the sunshine.
- Walk the dog at a slower pace for 30 minutes.
- House and yard work. You need to do these chores anyway; why not use them to break up work periods at the computer, or desk, exercise large muscle groups, and clear your mind?

Creating the time it takes to reduce stress is equally as crucial as these spur-of-the-moment breaks. If you set aside time to mentally and physically prepare yourself for the day, or to unwind at the end of a stressful day, you will have something to look forward to every day. I promise that if you make this time, you will begin to look forward to it each day as your renewal period. It will become a well-deserved "me time". You will come to protect it as an essential part of your day, and miss it when you don't take the time to de-stress.

During this stress reduction time that you set aside for yourself, you can exercise or engage in some other form of stress reduction. Here are some great activities that require little skill or preparation:

- Mediation
- Tai Chi
- Yoga
- Stretching exercises
- Motivational or inspirational reading (remember, it does not have to be physical, but nourishing the mind can also reduce symptoms of physical stress).

Meditation

Meditation is a factor in improving the function of the immune system. Studies conducted at the University of Wisconsin have confirmed this fact.

The study used a meditation technique called mindfulness-based stress reduction. Forty-eight healthy people were divided into two groups. They received meditation training for eight weeks and, in addition, received a vaccine for influenza.

Evaluation of blood samples at the fourth and eight-week mark indicated increased antibodies of significant levels, in the patients practicing the mediation techniques. This increase suggests that meditation helped to support the immune system, in becoming stronger and healthier. A healthy immune system is central to enjoying overall good health.

There are meditation techniques that you can use at any time, in any place. However, the most effective meditative practice, to relieve mental and physical stress, is when you can devote a specific amount of time to remove yourself from all external disruptions.

It does not have to take up much time, perhaps only 15 to 20 minutes, but it should be a quiet time, in a place where other people or the telephone cannot disturb you.

Mindfulness-Based Stress Reduction

The Mindfulness-Based Stress Reduction Technique (MBSR) for meditation was developed at the University of Massachusetts Medical Center in 1979. It is still widely practiced and regarded as effective today.

Proponents of MBSR, after more than 20 years of research, have concluded that the results can cover everything from an increased ability to relax, to improved self-esteem. They have also witnessed long-term reductions in physical and psychological symptoms.

The technique works, first by increasing awareness in all aspects of the individual. This includes a sense of your physical being and mental self. It is based on the premise that we already have this knowledge of self but must bring it to a point of awareness.

MBSR is credited with helping those who suffer from chronic pain or illness, headaches, high blood pressure, sleep and intestinal problems, along with anxiety disorders. It also benefits those who struggle with stress connected to work, the home or financial difficulties. These external stresses can lead to physical health problems that are able be alleviated, by practicing MBSR.

The technique works by being mindful of the sounds surrounding you, including your breathing. It focuses on rhythms and patterns, related to how we react to specific situations. The method includes stretching exercises, that help you achieve a mindful and aware state of being.

Acupuncture

This ancient Chinese method of inserting delicate needles into the body, to induce a physiological response, is more than 4,000 years old. It relates directly to the idea of so many other alternative medicines, including chiropractic, that the body has energy running through it. In Chinese, this energy is referred to as "Qi," and is pronounced as "*chee*." Qi has a direct impact on the balance and wellness of all systems found in the body.

Just like with nerve signals, Qi can have interference which prevents optimal health. The acupuncturist's goal is to remove these obstacles, just like the chiropractor removes a subluxation. Perhaps that is why many chiropractors also incorporate acupuncture, or the non-invasive, massage-like form of acupressure into their practice.

Acupuncture also has a body map, where specific stimulus points are related to various organs and systems. Sometimes acupuncture needles are inserted with a small electrical impulse, to stimulate the area further and remove the interference.

The energy is believed to flow down pathways called "meridians". The meridians need to be free from interference or obstructions, and in balance to achieve optimal health.

Tai Chi

Tai Chi is all about balance and harmony in the body and goes very well with chiropractic health care, as both strive for achieving that balance.

The balanced state within Tai Chi is often referred to as "Yin" and "Yang". The premise behind both Tai Chi and Chinese medicine is to increase the natural energy found in the body. In chiropractic, we refer to that natural energy as innate intelligence. When Chi is not flowing correctly in the body, there is a feeling of being unwell. Conversely, a free-flowing Chi within oneself leads to a sense of well-being.

Tai Chi can be considered both a physical and mental exercise. To awaken or release energy flow, specific movements and positions are enacted. Breathing techniques and exercises go hand in hand with the movements. These form sets and activities have different purposes, but all improve muscle tone, balance, flexibility, and mobility. They also work to improve concentration, by releasing a greater energy flow.

Tai Chi can be done at home, with videos to guide you. There are more and more classes and schools specific to the Chinese methods turning up, as people become more knowledgeable about the art. It has become more accepted as a viable method of maintaining good health.

Yoga

Yoga has many different applications for good health. There are specific movements, called poses, which can help with blood pressure, insomnia, osteoporosis and stress management. There are dozens of poses known to help with even more ailments and their prevention.

To perform yoga, the only "equipment" you need is an open mind and perhaps a good foam mat. This helps make some of the poses more comfortable. Loose clothing won't restrict your movements and is also essential.

There are several poses in Yoga which are explicitly designed for stress reduction. The following is a list of the common ones, by their English name.

Stress-Reducing Yoga Poses

Pose	Purpose/Benefit
Salutation Seal	Induces a state of meditation
Child's Pose	Suitable for returning to a restful, balanced state between other movements
Bharadvaja's Twist	Serves as a "tonic" to cleanse the abdominal organs and nourish the spine
Cobra Pose	It helps with spinal flexibility and opens the chest

Plow Pose	Used to reduce backache and promotes sound sleep
Noose Pose	Good for releasing tension
Supported Headstand	It has a calming effect on the brain and strengthens the whole body
Corpse Pose	A state of total relaxation is achieved
Bridge Pose	Rejuvenates tired legs
Standing Forward Bend	It soothes the mind and stretches the hamstrings
Extended Triangle Pose	The central standing pose for yoga is to center yourself

Each pose in Yoga can be challenging to achieve, the first few times you give it a try. It may seem to require a lot of effort and hardly be capable of reducing stress. Trying to clasp your hands behind your back might create more stress than it relieves, but each yoga pose is achievable with time and practice. With every session, there will be more and more flexibility and ease in completing the pose. As this happens more of your mind can release its attention from focusing on the movement, and the strain it seems to cause at first. Sticking with the program you will be able to realize its great stress-reducing benefits in just a few short weeks.

CHAPTER 7

THE NERVOUS SYSTEM CENTRAL TO GOOD HEALTH

When we were first conceived, the first thing created in all of us was the brain. Next, it was carefully encased in a bony hard substance called the cranium. Afterwards, the spinal cord, an extension of the brain, was created and that too was encased in a protective layer called the vertebrae, or spinal column.

The next part to be developed in-utero was the spinal nerve roots, which are extensions of the spinal cord. Ultimately, those spinal nerve roots create spinal nerves which are surrounded by embryonic tissue. The brain is then stimulated by the embryonic tissue via the superhighway called the nervous system. It was then and only then, that the other systems in the body developed.

You see, the nervous system is what controls all the systems in the body. If you were to look up the nervous system in Webster's Dictionary, you would find it defined as the following: "The master control system of the body that controls all other systems of the body."

The nervous system consists of three different areas. The first is the brain. It is the originator of the messages that are needed to be distributed to all the cells, tissues, organs, and systems of the body.

The second part of the nervous system is the spinal cord. Think of it as the superhighway of the nervous system. It is a complex system which has routes to every aspect of our body. The third part of the nervous system is the spinal nerve. Think of this as an exit off the main highway. Without these exits, you can never really get to a specific destination.

The brain weighs only 3 pounds. It needs only the energy of a 10-watt bulb, yet the functions of the brain are truly staggering. The brain is so complete and complex in its function that you would need two buildings the size of the Empire State Building to house today's technology that would rival the power of the brain.

Let me explain further. The brain can perform billions of operations simultaneously. Billions! A computer can only perform one task at a time. A computer can perform the task at astounding speeds, but it can only perform one function at a time. Therefore, in order to have the computer be able to replicate the full capacity of the nervous system, you would need a massive system enabling the computer to perform complex tasks; billions of them at the same time. That is why the nervous system is called the master control system of the body. It controls all other systems. Without it, you could not survive.

Here is another way to emphasize the importance of the nervous system. If you cut the nerve to the lungs, how would the lung know what to do? Think of the lung as an appliance, and the spinal cord is the circuit. If the circuit breaker isn't allowing energy to flow into the outlet that supplies the appliance, the appliance is not going to work. It's the same with the cells, tissues, organs, and systems of the body.

The Workings of the Nervous System

Intelligence flows through every cell in the body. This intelligence is referred to by chiropractors as Innate Intelligence. Without this intelligence, there would be no order and no divine collaboration within our body.

There is an internal divine guidance that guides all the functions of the body. It knows exactly what substance to produce at the exact time needed. The neuronal connections within our body are truly staggering. In the brain alone, there are more possible connections than there are possible combinations of phone lines within the United States. Just imagine that number!

So, what prevents our body from doing its thing? What prevents this splendid orchestra from playing its tune called health?

Interference with the nervous system can have serious complications. Think about this for a moment. If I'm on a phone and I'm giving you very detailed instructions on how to get from point A to point B, and all of a sudden your phone begins to break up, will you be able to accurately get the directions you need to get to your destination? Now, this is not because you are incompetent. It is simply due to the fact that there was a break in your communication with me.

The key is to maintain 100 % communication within every aspect of the body. The researchers are just beginning to understand that there are mechanisms within our bodies that are trying to communicate something very important. One example is the fever. At first, fever was regarded as something that needed to be stopped. We now know that it is designed to throw off foreign invaders.

How did we react to fevers just 10 years ago? We pushed fever-reducing substances down our children's throats, and we bought into it. There are so many examples of this type of message scrambling that we do to ourselves, be it emotionally, physically, nutritionally, etc. Misunderstandings take place all the time. That is why I'm writing this book - to at least give you a basic understanding of your body and what you can do immediately to bring it to the next level. You have a very sophisticated body which needs a sophisticated understanding of how to provide it with the essential care it needs.

If the entire nervous system is fully functioning and fully interactive, with all the cells, tissues, organs, and other systems in the body, then the body can effectively and efficiently respond appropriately to dangerous conditions in the body. However, if the nervous system is not functioning properly, then you will find that it will create an imbalance, or lack of ease also called dis-ease.

The mindset that we have regarding our bodies must be changed. Do we just get by in a cruel world, or is life a miracle, and the body that I am in the temple of my soul? Do we have reverence for our bodies? Again, this book is a wake-up call for you to realize that there is so much in all of us to stimulate health - so much potential. Unfortunately, most of the time, through ignorance, the body is just wasted away.

In the coming chapters, you will realize that our bodies can be the most amazing source of super immuno-stimulation and yet it can also be the greatest source of disease creation. The great researcher Gary Null has advocated that health can be broken down into 25% nutrition, 25% exercising, and a whopping 50% mental attitude. If we have certain expectations and we believe them with certainty, those expectations will manifest in the physical world. In other words, you truly become what you think about, good or bad. What we must remember is that the intelligence that created us at conception still flows through every cell in our body today, and we must honour that.

The body is providing us with signals, and we can not ignore those signals. Again, I will stress one thing; I, or any other chiropractor, doctor or naturopath do not cure anything or anyone! The body does the curing. If any healthcare provider truly understood the innate intelligence that flows through us all, he or she would humbly become obedient to that intelligence and do everything they could to align themselves with the principles of health.

The body can either be used in its amazing splendour or it can be abused, and if it is abused, you will suffer the consequences of natural law. So, if we are to attain incredible levels of health, we must first start with an equivalent level of gratitude for our body and respect for it. When you realize that you have a choice, to make this life what you want of it, to carve out of life what you want, to create a magical life full of passion, vibrancy, and possibility, then you must be grateful for what you have.

Think about it. There are so many things for which you can and should be grateful. The body that you are in right now is doing everything it can to support you at this very moment. It is there to serve you. So today I want you to decide that from now on, you will no longer look at your body as something that deserves a candy bar or a soda. Think of it as one of the finest, exotic cars in the world, one that deserves and should receive only the best fuel.

If you owned a $100,000 racehorse, you would train it constantly. You would feed it the best food possible. Why? Because you paid all that money, and you expect to get a return on your investment. Well, what do you suppose you and your health are worth? How much would you be willing to pay for a liver transplant? How much for a kidney transplant? How much for a heart transplant? How much for your hearing? How much for your vision?

Can you now see how valuable and priceless you really are?

Realize that you are a gift from your creator and that you are here for a reason. That you are here not to be a wandering generality, but a meaningful specific, a person destined to achieve something worthwhile.

You can't attain your heart's desires without the spark of energy derived from a true level of health and well-being. Begin today with a new appreciation that your life demands true energy, not just bouts of it. It deserves a level of health that rivals the idea you once thought of as acceptable.

CHAPTER 8

THE SPINE

The spine is composed of the spinal cord, discs, nerves, and vertebrae, all of which are central to the techniques and science of chiropractic. The spinal column is a row of bones that encircles the spinal cord, protecting it while also regulating its range of motion. The spinal cord is the main part of the central nervous system, which transmits signals throughout the body. The spinal cord and the nerves found there only transmit signals concerning touch and feelings of pain.

The nerves send signals of pain when you experience an accident or injury. This pain is registered in the brain, which then instructs the body to react quickly to avoid the source of that pain. For example, when you burn your hand on the stove and jerk it away quickly! Though this is correct, there is much more to the information and signals sent from the nervous system to the brain and other organs in the body, which are deeply connected to how our organs and overall system functions.

In chiropractic, it is known that every area of the body is supplied with vital information from the nerves. Chiropractors remove any cases of subluxation through adjustments or manipulations, allowing every organ to function at its highest capacity. This is the number one purpose of chiropractic: to remove static disruption between the brain and the rest of the body, opening up channels for it to heal and mend via its innate intelligence.

Regions of the Spine

The spine can be broken down into three key regions: the cervical, thoracic, and lumbar regions. There is also a fourth area referred to as the sacral region; however, this region only has two bones — the sacrum and the coccyx — found at the bottom of the spine and extending into the pelvic area. The vertebrae are numbered within the top three regions of the spine. Thus, when there is a misalignment in a particular vertebra, the chiropractor can explain and show the patient that a misalignment of the C4 vertebra is the cause of the issue. This would mean that the fourth vertebra in the cervical spine is misaligned.

A patient with a blockage or misalignment of the C4 vertebra could end up seeing their doctor for hay fever and not necessarily for back pain. That is because the nerves that extend from the C4 vertebra are responsible for sending messages to the nose, lips, mouth, Eustachian tube, and mucous membranes. Oftentimes, a misalignment may manifest itself as symptoms related to hay fever, postnasal drips, adenoid infections, and other upper respiratory difficulties. Even problems with one's hearing can develop due to a misalignment of the C4 vertebra.

Every nerve extending from the spinal column is responsible for an organ, a function, or a performance of some body part. These include the more apparent perceptions, such as touch, which are connected to all other aspects of the body. If you envision an outline of the body and draw lines out from the vertical centerline where the spine is located to each extremity, you can see how the nerves spread out and connect to many areas of the body. Imagine, then, how important a proper alignment of the vertebrae, which are meant to protect the spinal cord and nerves, is and what the effect may be on too many organs and bodily functions if this is pushed slightly out of place, or the nerves in the spine are left pinched or squeezed?

How the Spine Moves

The spine can bend, move, twist, and return to its "S"-like shape without incident or injury due to the soft tissue and parts that work in conjunction with the bony vertebrae. Two areas are essential in helping the spinal column protect the large mass of nerve tissue running through it.

One part is the intervertebral discs, which can be found between each vertebra. These discs help absorb shock and impact as the spine bends and twists during normal movement and activity. This is not something one thinks about when bending down to pick up a toy off the floor, as everything is in its proper place and functioning correctly. You can bend and twist to one side, grasping the toy that slid under the chair, without incurring any physical problems. However, if you were to have a deterioration in one of those discs, or if it were to have slipped out of place, even slightly, the bones in the spine could grind together, pinching a nerve, which would cause you to feel pain.

The second part is the facet joints, which allow for limited movement of the spine and help regulate the range of motion so that routine movements are restricted up to a certain point, thus helping to prevent any injury to the spine that might otherwise be caused by excessive stress or overload.

Misaligned Vertebrae

Every nerve in the body radiating out from the spinal cord supplies essential information to its respective area of the body, which it is responsible for. The example of the C4 vertebra being out of alignment is just one possible outcome of hundreds of slight misalignments that can cause subluxation and interfere with important nerve signals, often resulting in various symptoms of illness or discomfort.

A patient visiting a traditional medical doctor because of indigestion issues or heartburn will often be prescribed a form of antacid to ease their uncomfortable symptoms. This type of quick fix may work for a while and can provide some immediate relief, but the problem with this approach is that it does not cure the actual health issue;

it hardly even addresses it, neglecting the real cause of the problem. How can the body ever hope to heal itself if medications are momentarily and constantly silencing symptoms?

Symptoms are there for a reason. The body, in its wisdom, is informing the brain that something is not right. If we silence that inner voice with drugs, it is like telling someone to stop talking when they are trying to warn you about an impending car. They are attempting to give you a significant message and if you ignore it long enough, you may eventually have to contend with a much more serious problem.

When there are any symptoms of illness related to the stomach, it can often be traced back to the T6 vertebrae, if the nerves in this region experience some kind of interference. Removing that blockage through an adjustment of the spine opens up the lines of communication to the stomach and allows for the problem in that area to be corrected naturally.

This simplified lesson on the anatomy of the spine is meant to illustrate the complexity of the spinal column and the importance of the spinal cord; however, it is much more complex than what is explained here. Many other unmentioned misalignments can impact different regions of the body in various ways. Symptoms may manifest themselves in different manners, and it can be difficult to pinpoint the actual cause.

Headaches, stomach aches, allergic reactions, asthma, nasal drips, and some types of hearing difficulties can originate from nerves connected to these areas, which are being compromised by a subluxation. Chiropractors have studied the complexities of the central nervous system, the musculoskeletal system, and the spine for years in order to perform proper diagnostic tests and serve their patients with the best treatment for many types of ailments and health issues.

CHAPTER 9

THE MISTAKES WE MAKE EVERYDAY

Each day, we make unconscious mistakes that put our spinal health and overall wellness at stake. Some of the most common ones can be found here as well as ways to correct or avoid making the same mistakes day after day.

From morning to night, there are small adjustments we can make to improve posture and protect our backs. These tips include all of the principles of ergonomics. They show simple and subtle ways we can reduce tension that leads to back trouble.

- Start the day off right with a good stretch. Hug your arms around yourself, and then turn to the left and the right.

Stretching in the morning can be one of the most beneficial activities you can do for your body each day. While it may not appear to be a major thing, stretching helps loosen tight muscles, improve posture and joint mobility, and even increase blood circulation throughout your body. It also helps reduce stress and tension that can accumulate over time.

It's best to do a few stretches each day, but don't overexert yourself or push too far into a stretch. Listen to your body and take it slow. You can start by incorporating simple neck and shoulder rolls, side bends, hip circles, ankle rotations, and more into your daily routine. As you increase the variety of stretches you do, remember that even gentle stretching can be effective in improving how you feel both physically and mentally.

So, give it a try! Taking just five minutes out of your morning for some stretching can make all the difference in how you approach your day.

- When brushing your teeth, don't hunch over the sink. Stand up straight, and bend at the waist when you need to rinse.

When brushing your teeth, maintaining good posture and avoiding slouching are important for your overall health and well-being. Keeping a good posture while brushing your teeth can help maintain proper alignment of your spine, as well as improve posture over time. Poor posture can lead to muscular imbalances, back pain, and other health issues in the long term.

When brushing your teeth, it is best to stand up straight and bend at the waist when you need to rinse. This is because it allows you to keep your back in its natural curvature, which helps prevent strain on the muscles and joints. It also keeps the head up so that you don't put too much pressure on one side of the neck or shoulders. When brushing, try not to hunch forward or lean on one side – make sure that you actively engage your core muscles so that you remain upright and balanced throughout the process.

Good posture is vital for overall health, as it helps to reduce fatigue, prevent muscle tension and aches and pains in areas like the neck, shoulder, and back. Additionally, standing upright while brushing encourages proper breathing habits which can help improve oxygenation throughout the body. Furthermore, standing upright with a good posture can give off a sense of confidence, helping you feel more positive about yourself!

Practicing good posture each day while brushing your teeth will become easier and more comfortable over time, providing both short-term and long-term benefits for your physical health and general well-being!

- Make sure the chairs are the right height and depth for your body. You should be able to sit back and still have 2 inches between the end of the chair and your knees. This will help you maintain a good posture.

When it comes to choosing the right chair for your body, it is important to ensure it is of the correct height and depth. A chair that is too low or too shallow can cause strain on the back, neck, and shoulders due to incorrect posture. Sitting in a chair that does not fit properly can result in long-term damage to the body and can even lead to chronic pain. It is essential to find a chair that fits comfortably against your back and leaves two inches between the end of the seat and your knees.

Having an appropriate height for your chair will help you maintain good posture, which is key in maintaining spinal health. Proper posture reduces the stress on joints and muscles, allowing them to move more freely without causing pain or discomfort. Muscles have a greater range of motion when seated in a chair with proper support, helping you stay comfortable while sitting for extended periods of time.

Properly-sized chairs also help reduce pressure on your spine; this helps prevent fatigue caused by slouching or hunching over while sitting in an uncomfortable position. When seated in a well-fitted chair, there is less strain on the lower back as your weight is distributed evenly throughout the seat. Additionally, having a correctly-sized chair encourages proper seating habits, such as keeping feet flat on the floor with legs bent at 90 degrees or slightly greater angles.

- Ensure that you have adequate lighting for all tasks, as one of the main causes of tension headaches is poor lighting and the associated eye strain.

Poor lighting can cause a number of ailments, with one of the most common being tension headaches. These headaches are caused by the muscles in your neck and scalp contracting too tightly, leading to a feeling of tightness or pressure around your head. Poor lighting, especially artificial lighting such as fluorescent and LED lights, not only causes eye strain but can also result in tension headaches.

When we don't have enough natural light entering our eyes, they become strained. Eye strain can cause discomfort and fatigue, which, in turn, can lead to tension headaches. Even when natural light is present, if optical conditions are still inadequate, then this will contribute to eye strain and create an uncomfortable environment in which to work or carry out activities. Many studies have found that the quality of light is just as important as its quantity; too much bright light, or flickering light, can lead to eyestrain and tension headaches.

An ideal lighting environment should be one in which the brightness levels are kept consistent throughout the day. Fluctuations between very bright and very dark environments can put additional stress on your eyes as well. Good lighting should also be free from glares; direct sunlight should not be allowed into windows or onto other surfaces within the workplace in order to avoid reflection glares from shiny screens, desks, or glass surfaces.

In order to avoid developing a tension headache, it is important to ensure that you have adequate lighting for any tasks you undertake. This way, your eyes won't suffer from unnecessary eyestrain and you'll remain comfortable while performing whatever task you are working on, with minimal risk of developing a tension headache as a result of poor lighting conditions!

- Avoid wearing high-heeled shoes, as they can cause spinal stress due to the uneven distribution of weight between the heel and toe.

High-heeled shoes can cause significant stress and tension on the spine, as the unnatural elevation of the heel causes an uneven distribution of weight between the heel and toe, putting the spine in an unnatural position. This may result in misalignment and micro-movements that can strain muscles and the ligaments attached to or near the spinal column.

Prolonged wear of high-heeled shoes can also lead to pain, discomfort, and instability in areas such as the lower back, neck, and shoulders. Additionally, when wearing high-heeled shoes for extended periods of time, it can cause a decrease in flexibility in these areas as well as increased tightness and stiffness.

In more severe cases, long-term use of high heels can cause permanent damage to the bones and tendons surrounding the spine due to the increased pressure on them over time. This could result in chronic pain that may persist even after quitting wearing such shoes. In some cases, even moderate use of high heels can cause disc herniation between vertebrae, as well as other forms of spinal trauma such as spondylolisthesis or muscle strain around spinal joints.

Overall, high-heeled shoes are not recommended for daily wear due to their negative impacts on spinal health over time. If you must wear them occasionally, try limiting their usage or wearing ones with a lower heel height (up to 2 inches). It is also important to take frequent breaks while wearing this type of footwear, so that your body has time to adjust and recover from any stress put on it by the elevated heel height. Finally, be sure to do a good stretch after wearing high-heeled shoes for a period of time; this will help alleviate any tension built up in your spine during use.

- Sitting with your legs crossed in the same direction can eventually lead to spinal misalignment. Ideally, both feet should be kept on the floor while sitting.

Sitting with your legs crossed in the same direction can cause a wide range of negative health issues, such as spinal misalignments, which can lead to back pain and increased stress on the muscles and joints. Over time, this poor posture may even result in permanent structural damage. Even if it doesn't cause severe health problems, it can still be uncomfortable and tiring!

When you sit cross-legged, you tend to lean forward, making it harder for your lower back to be properly supported. This causes you to slouch, leading to a decrease in support for your spinal column. Inadequate support for the lower back makes it more susceptible to strain from repetitive motion or incorrect posture. Your risk of developing muscle fatigue or pain increases significantly when sitting with your legs crossed for extended periods of time.

Crossing your legs also places additional strain on the hip flexors and external rotators of the hip joint, which can lead to tightness and discomfort in those areas over time. Sitting with your legs crossed may also push the pelvis out of alignment, causing further tension in other areas of the body, such as the calves or hamstrings, and impede circulation in the lower extremities. To protect yourself from any potential negative effects associated with sitting cross-legged, it is important that you keep both feet on the floor while sitting and maintain proper spinal alignment throughout your body while seated.

- Holding a telephone receiver with your shoulder can cause the spinal joints to lock up in the upper back, neck, and shoulders. Use your hand or a headset if you need to have your hands free.

Holding a phone with your shoulder can cause the spinal joints to lock up in the upper back, neck, and shoulders. This can lead to tension headaches, neck pain and discomfort, as well as restricted range of motion in those body parts and their surrounding joint structures, over time.

Additionally, this also adds further stress and strain from the weight of the device itself. When straining your neck muscles for long periods of time during phone calls, or even conversations with friends or family members on social media apps, this can cause inflammation in the nearby muscles and tendons which may lead to chronic problems over time.

The incorrect posture associated with holding a smartphone up against your chin or shoulder can also create imbalances within the spine that might not be noticed until it is too late. Over time this imbalance will lead to further issues such as pinched nerves which may cause tingling sensations radiating down limbs, numbness and limited mobility throughout the entire body due to tightness in specific areas such as hips, lower back and hamstrings.

- If you have a desk job, be sure to get up and move around frequently. It is important to change positions often, especially if you are sitting while doing repetitive motions, such as typing at a computer.

Sitting at a desk in front of a computer for hours on end can have a detrimental effect on one's health. An overly sedentary lifestyle is associated with higher risks of obesity, cardiovascular diseases, and diabetes. Studies have shown that those who do not get enough physical activity are more likely to suffer from chronic diseases and ailments.

That's why it is so important to take regular breaks from sitting and get some movement in. Take a few minutes every hour to stand up, stretch your body, and walk around the office. Alternatively, you could try doing some simple exercises like squats or lunges at your desk; these will help improve your posture, range of motion, and overall health.

A yoga chair can be a great way to promote good spinal health while working at a desk. Unlike traditional chairs, the ergonomic design of a yoga chair allows for greater movement and flexibility while sitting, thus promoting relaxation and good posture. The sloped seat encourages users to sit up straight in order to maintain correct positioning, thereby helping improve back and neck alignment.

- Find ways to reduce emotional stress and tension; that will carry over into your posture if left to fester.

Chronic stress is a major health concern in today's world, and it can have serious, negative effects on both physical and mental health. Prolonged exposure to stress can increase blood pressure, cholesterol levels, and heart rates as well as weaken the immune system, making the body more susceptible to various illnesses and diseases. Chronic stress has been linked to depression and anxiety. Emotional stress can also cause hormonal imbalances, as well as changes in sleep patterns, making it difficult for the body to recover from strenuous activities or repair itself from sickness or injury. Furthermore, chronic emotional stress can lead to fatigue, headaches, and muscle tension due to prolonged periods of tense muscles.

More alarmingly, studies have shown that prolonged periods of emotional stress can increase a person's risk for developing conditions such as diabetes, obesity, and hypertension. This is because emotional stress triggers a fight-or-flight response in the body, releasing cortisol, the primary hormone involved in this response. Cortisol increases blood sugar levels, putting strain on the cardiovascular system over time and potentially leading to long-term damage.

Achieving a good work-life balance is essential for one's overall health and well-being. When one lives a balanced life with enough time to both work and play, it can lead to improved physical and well-being. Studies have shown that individuals who manage their work and leisure activities in a healthy manner demonstrate an increased sense of satisfaction and fulfillment. They are also less likely to experience fatigue, depression, or anxiety. Creating a healthy work-life balance can help to reduce stress levels and improve overall physical health. It also allows people to find the time for regular exercise, which supports greater heart health.

Additionally, having regular breaks throughout the day gives individuals the opportunity to rest and relax as needed, helping them stay focused on task completion during their working hours and improving their overall productivity levels.

- Get plenty of sleep on a quality mattress and a good pillow that supports the neck and spine.

A quality mattress and a good pillow that support the spine are essential for getting a restful night's sleep. Not only do these ensure comfort, but they also help to alleviate many health problems associated with lack of sleep or sleeping on an inadequate mattress or pillow.

A spine-friendly pillow helps to promote healthy spinal alignment by providing support for the neck, shoulders, and head while sleeping. It can help reduce pressure points in the shoulder and neck area that may cause pain due to poor posture during sleep. This reduces the chances of developing musculoskeletal problems, such as stiff necks, headaches, muscle tension, and joint pain. A spine-friendly pillow also ensures adequate lumbar support, thus helping to maintain proper back posture during sleep. This prevents fatigue caused by poor body alignment which can lead to chronic back pain over time if not addressed properly.

Good sleep quality has been linked to improved focus and concentration levels throughout the day. With a supportive pillow designed specifically for the spine, the body is kept in its natural position during rest, which allows for adequate oxygen flow throughout the body, resulting in better quality sleep with fewer disturbances throughout the night. Having enough restful nights increases energy levels during daily activities and may even help improve moods, since there are fewer aches and pains associated with poor posture when sleeping on an inferior mattress or pillow.

CHAPTER 10

THE PIERCE RESULTS SYSTEM & SPECIFIC CHIROPRACTIC ADJUSTMENTS

Dr. Walter V. Pierce designed the Pierce Results System over his 30+ year career. His goal was to take the best chiropractic had to offer, improve upon and add to it, and create the best system of spinal care the world had ever seen. With the use of state-of-the-art "Video fluoroscopy" (spinal video scans), "Digital Infrared Thermal Imaging" (digital nerve scans), and the most advanced manual and computerized adjusting techniques, he did just that!

Before any spinal adjustment occurs, a chiropractor will assess the patient with specific diagnostic tools. One such tool is spinal palpation, a test where the chiropractor uses physical touch to evaluate the degree of mobility of the spine, along with any possible malfunctions.

Spinal palpation can be performed as a static or motion palpation. In static palpation, the chiropractor assesses by touch while the patient is still. This primarily tests for sensitivity, pain, or any swelling in areas of the spine.

This tactile diagnostic method is used with visual images, taken from X-rays or other imaging tests.

Motion palpation does just what the term implies – measures motion. A joint is naturally capable of a certain degree of motion, and then there is the "end-play". End-play is the absolute limit to the range of motion, that extra bit of flexibility that the spine is capable of after the natural stopping point of the joint. The degree of end-play, with or without pain, is vital in any diagnostic assessment.

Unfortunately, studies show motion palpation is unreliable in assessing spinal joint mobility. While we still utilize static and motion palpation at our clinic, we must offer the gold standard and best that chiropractic offers for joint motion assessment. For this reason, we have committed to providing Joint Motion Imaging (JMI) in all appropriate clinical circumstances. Our current JMI suite has a video fluoroscopy (VF) machine.

This machine utilizes small dose radiation with an image-intensifying tube to see the spine in live motion. While this technology is still the gold standard, new developments are happening every day, and we are committed to making sure our JMI technology is always up-to-date.

Specific Adjustments to Handle a Subluxation

Adjusting the spine through specific movements of the vertebrae is one of the most effective ways of handling a subluxation. Subluxation is a slight misalignment of vertebrae and loss of normal spinal joint motion that prevents nerves from sending clear, uninterrupted signals between the brain and various parts of the body, which over time, can lead to several forms of illness and disorders.

The term disease is broken down to the coined word "dis-ease" in chiropractic terminology. This implies a reduction in wellness instead of the medical term, which indicates a health issue or an illness. In chiropractic, the focus is on general wellness and a whole-body approach to treating illnesses, disorders, or any health issues, in cooperation with the body's innate intelligence. Innate intelligence is the inborn, natural force found in any organism that helps maintain a healthy state. This allows the body to operate at its highest capacity and seeks to return a patient to a balanced state, known as "homeostasis."

That Cracking Sound

The "popping" sound many people hear during an adjustment at the chiropractor is called "cavitation." It is the release of nitrogen gasses from the synovial fluid in the joint, and it is painless and harmless in the hands of a trained chiropractor. It is a reaction that enables the joint to move more freely and aids in releasing toxins from the body.

Types of Adjustments

Earlier in chiropractic, spinal adjustments were almost solely based on a pure hands-on approach to adjusting the vertebrae to handle a subluxation. The amount of pressure, the angle of the movements, and the positioning of the hands were the primary methods for varying the force of the adjustment.

During an adjustment, traditional hands-on techniques and adjusting instruments can be utilized. Both approaches are very effective, and these days, most chiropractors use several types of techniques for many types of patients and circumstances.

Using only a couple of fingers and a very gentle approach by a trained professional, even newborns can receive a spinal adjustment and benefit from it.

Pierce Results System (PRS) Adjustments

Terminal Point Drop Adjustments

This may be the most common adjustment technique, even for those new to chiropractic or who may have a preconceived notion of what a visit to the chiropractor entails. During a table adjustment, the patient lies down on a special table. Quick thrusts are applied to specific areas of the spine, and the table is designed to drop slightly simultaneously with the thrusts of the adjustment. This assists with the speed and effectiveness of the adjustment. This is a gentler method than a typical manual adjustment as it bypasses the body's natural guarding mechanisms, and less pressure is needed to get the spine to move.

Instrument Adjustments

Instrument-based adjustments are utilized with several types of techniques, including PRS. An early example of these instruments is the "activator," a spring-loaded, mechanical device that is gentle and effective. Certain types of chiropractic techniques can thus be applied to children, the elderly, or patients who are otherwise fragile or in greater pain levels.

Newer types of instruments that use computerized impulses are also available. Our office has a particular type of multiple-impulse instrument called a "PulStar G3". The G3 is a vibrational impulse instrument that can send up to 50 impulses per second into the desired segment of the spine or associated structures. It can provide speed, reproducibility, and accuracy in its application toward subluxation removal – it can also read the patient's response in real time while adjusting the instrument's frequency to best complement each person individually.

CHAPTER 11

DIAGNOSTIC METHODS USED IN CHIROPRACTIC

A typical patient evaluation and history taking at a chiropractic office are similar to that of a traditional visit to a medical doctor. Chiropractors are also trained in using various diagnostic tools that can hone in on and differentiate between several health problems or issues.

Some of the standard tests used in chiropractic are orthopedic and neurological in nature. This pertains to X-rays, ultrasound, range of motion and mobility analysis. There is also a hands-on type of examination, where a trained chiropractor can feel obvious misalignments present in the spine when vertebrae have shifted to the point where it causes interference with the neurological signals transmitted by the radiating nerves.

Several diagnostic instruments are used by chiropractors. Many of these, in their earliest form, were used by B.J. Palmer, the father of chiropractic himself. Their modern versions are equally as effective in targeting misalignments and the resulting subluxations. Some cutting-edge technological advancements have also been brought to light by the growing field of chiropractic. Working with tried-and-true instruments and the newest technology allows chiropractors to get a more complete picture of the situation, before recommending and beginning any kind of care.

Subluxation Stations

There is a kind of instrument used in chiropractic that offers a complete look and analysis of where and what kind of subluxation is taking place in the patient. It uses a static surface electromyogram (sEMG) to measure electrical activity and creates a color map of sorts that shows where muscular imbalance is taking place.

Another colorful illustration seen is the result of the kind of thermal activity which is taking place in the muscles, tissues, and skin around the spine. It can show a measurement of paraspinal infrared temperatures, to automatically measure the balance in the autonomic (or subconscious) branch of the peripheral nervous system. Pain thresholds and heart rate variability (HRV), a technology that also maps autonomic balance, can also be measured along the spine with a subluxation station.

Thermal Imaging Instruments

First used in chiropractic in 1924, thermal technology has been used by health practitioners for over a century. Digital infrared thermal imaging (DITI) uses infrared technology to non-invasively assess the function of the autonomic nerve system. This is the involuntary part of the nerve system that tells your heart to beat, stomach to digest, and liver to produce enzymes vital for everyday life, to name but a few! Experts like neurosurgeon Dr. Jose Ochoa have called DITI,

"...the most valuable test available for evaluating the autonomic nerve system."

Dr. Jaszewski is one of only a few in New Jersey and the country with this powerful technology.

Infrared imaging is used to view changes in temperature where soft-tissue injuries may have occurred. A process called Computerized Infrared Thermography (CIT) is also implemented by the use of a handheld paraspinal scanner. One such instrument called the "TyTron" has been developed by Titronics Research and Development, in Iowa City, IA. The device scans and generates graphs that can be laid out, one over the other, for analysis and comparison.

Video fluoroscopy (Joint Motion Imaging)

If you were a detective… and you could choose between having pictures of a crime scene or video footage of the crime taking place – which would you choose?? The video of course! This is one of the most important contributions Dr. Walter V. Pierce gave to the chiropractic profession – the ability to SEE spinal problems instead of just "feeling" them. Research shows this new technology increases the accuracy of detecting spinal misalignments chiropractors refer to as "subluxations" up to 93%!!! Dr. Jaszewski is one of only a handful of chiropractors in New Jersey and the country with this new technology.

The Nervo-Scope

This instrument was developed by the Virginia-based company, Electronic Development Labs, and is used both before and after a chiropractor makes any adjustments to a patient's spine. Before the manipulation, the scope assesses temperature readings taken along the spine. Following the adjustment, the readings are again recorded, to measure the difference. This allows the chiropractor to observe the degree of reduction in subluxation that has occurred.

The Myogauge

This trademarked instrument created by the Myogauge Corp., in Deer Park, NY, primarily measures the range of motion and isometric muscle strength for any part of the body. The systems are highly customized, so each practitioner can add the accessories that best serve their patients. The computerized system documents result from digitally measuring the amount of force created by the patient's movements.

Regional Spinal Testing

There are instruments used in chiropractic that focus on the various regions of the spinal column, which measure and record results in the form of impulse response and a waveform created by the spine.

Dr. Jaszewski utilizes the PulStar G3 instrument from Sense Technologies. The G3 is a vibrational impulse instrument that can send up to 50 impulses per second into the desired segment of the spine or associated structures. Not only can it provide speed, reproducibility, and accuracy in its application toward subluxation removal – it can also read the patient's response in real time while adjusting the frequency of the instrument to best complement each person individually.

Other instruments used in spinal screening incorporate bilateral weight and postural evaluations. This is the case with the Rapid Posture Imaging system (SAM), developed by the S.A.M. Company of Henderson, NV.

The explanation of these complex technologies, which is associated with chiropractic methods of diagnosis, is to illustrate the advances that have been made. A visit to the chiropractor is not the cliché bone-cracking session often envisioned, based on a hit-or-miss assessment.

The spine is one of the most important, if not *the* most important, system in the body. No legitimate, well-trained, or educated chiropractor is going to proceed with any adjustments or manipulations in the dark! Sophisticated instrumentation and diagnostic tools are constantly emerging. These are available for chiropractors to make educated evaluations and precise adjustments in their treatment plans, after which they are then able to adequately document the progress in healing.

These diagnostic tools are expertly used to diagnose a wide range of misalignments, or issues, which could prevent complete wellness. They are designed to spot a potential problem long before the patient ever experiences any symptoms!

CHAPTER 12

PHASES OF HEALING

This chapter is dedicated to describing specific phases of healing, to better explain how increasing your strength, health, and longevity can be approached. But first, let me clarify something: Chiropractic care is not a quick fix or an overnight miracle. If your system is currently out of balance, then it is certain that other issues have been present for a long time, which have led to the development of any unhealthy condition you are presently experiencing. The good news is that it will most likely not take you years to regain your health, but it may take some time.

Therefore, you need to practice patience and devotion. Let's now go over the phases of healing, one after the other.

STAGE 1 - THE INTENSE INFLAMMATORY PHASE

This is a phase where people are encouraged to pay more attention to their health and to seek expert help. It could be with conventional medicine, or by alternative means, and most forms of pain experienced in this phase are governed by discomfort.

Chiropractic methods are not painful. What triggers the sensation of pain is your system's reaction to the state of sore tissue and muscles, or pinched nerves signaling pain through the body when the chiropractor works on them. If your body has been subjected to inflammation, pain, or other health issues for a prolonged period, then it may be more sensitive to pain than a healthy body.

This is the stage where patients often see the chiropractor with complaints of pain or signs of discomfort, such as swelling, soreness, aches, stiffness, or a loss of balance. Oftentimes patients at this stage do not see us because they want to improve their health, but because they are fed up with being in pain or discomfort. Their main concern is to reduce their pain and to seek relief – not the underlying mechanics, which may be the cause of their issue.

It needs to be emphasized that the body does not arrive at this stage overnight. It takes years to reach such a painful state: Years of mishandling and inappropriate movement, stress, and strain. Therefore, healing during this initial stage may also require some time, and you might have to visit a chiropractor's office once or twice a week, for a while. Although this may sound a bit exaggerated to the average person seeking a quick fix, it is in reality a small investment in your long-term health.

It should be noted that therapy can vary regarding power and frequency, based on the following factors:

- Sex
- Age
- Height
- Weight
- The time you've been suffering from the health issue
- The degree you can follow your physician's direction
- The amount of pain you can tolerate
- If you are experiencing other health problems

At the initial consultation, the chiropractor will assess all of the above parameters, and any other relevant aspects or problems, to be able to design a personalized plan for your care. Your personal needs and challenges are also considered, and anyone chiropractic approach may not be the same for everyone.

STAGE 2 - THE RESTORATIVE AND CORRECTIVE STAGE

During this phase, your pain and discomfort begin to subside. Your pain will become more tolerable and although you may not feel as if you are progressing at lightning speeds, you will experience much less discomfort and have a more positive attitude toward your health.

We rely on this phase, to rehabilitate strength, and integrity and to stabilize the patient on the road to full recovery. This is an excellent stage as the patient begins to experience betterment. Energy levels increase, discomfort is greatly minimized, and the range of motion is restored. As pain "eats" away vast amounts of energy, the level of pain reduction and boosting of energy levels can be quite remarkable, at this stage.

However, there is one aspect that we need to pay extra attention to during this phase, to avoid pushing or forcing the patient too much. When most people begin to feel better under treatment, they might mistakenly think themselves able to do much more than they really can. The dilemma is in pushing yourself too hard, too early, and causing strain or inappropriate stress, which can result in renewed damage or setbacks.

During this phase, our aim in chiropractic is to concentrate focus on boosting spinal mobility, so that healthy physiological function is restored to your spine and nerves. You might still have to visit your chiropractor once a week, but it all depends on the intensity of your condition.

Keep in mind that this corrective stage is not usually brief, and that other parameters and factors affect the speed of healing. If you for example come to the office after having suffered multiple car accidents in a row, it will most likely require more time for the treatments to take a noticeable effect, compared to the average patient who is simply dealing with a poor posture. Some of the following things affect treatment and slow down progress:

- A poor diet, or lacking nutrition
- Smoking
- Stress
- Improper ergonomics
- A negative mindset

STAGE 3 – THE MAINTENANCE STAGE

I love having patients at this specific stage visit me. Arriving at this stage means that they have followed the treatment directions and that they are doing what they can, to restore their health and well-being. Pain is greatly minimized at this stage, or at least kept under control and managed.

Once the body achieves a state of good health, it is necessary to maintain it. However, keeping your body healthy is much easier at this phase. Remember that a state of perfect health does not just imply a lack of pain and disease - it is a state of optimal physical, mental, and personal well-being.

Another advantage of the body arriving at this stage of health is that it will have a better ability to recover if you incur any accidents in the future, and intense treatment will no longer be necessary. When highly practiced and fit athlete experiences an injury, they are usually able to recover quicker than the average person. This is because they are used to conditioning practice and their system is at an optimal state of health. Recovery is therefore much faster!

Consider kids and the rate at that they often recover from injuries. This is because our system is designed to recover and restore health quickly, from a very young age. As we grow older, the rate of recovery deteriorates, and we are often less resistant and less able to fight off health issues.

This stage goes further than regular chiropractic care, however. It comes down to lifelong habits and health patterns. This is the point where people may experience a certain degree of discomfort, as they transition to a healthier diet, start to exercise more, and build a positive, stress-free mindset.

Often excuses stand in the way of this point, with one of the classic ones being a lack of sufficient time to exercise, prepare healthy food or ensure good sleep. There is always time to decide on what is essential for a good quality of life and to make that your priority. You must take care of your health, in your way.

Nathaniel Branden, an inspiring psychologist who has written several books on self-confidence and self-esteem, believes that the things we try to improve are the things we have already realized are flawed, while the areas we neglect to work on are the ones we ignore, and which we feel are beyond our control. This also applies to our health. You must work on it every day, and you will become able to efficiently work towards its achievement once you have the necessary means.

People tend to make this step overly complicated, but here are a few questions you can use to help improve your health:

- How can I enjoy eating properly today and working out?
- What foods can I eat that are healthy and delicious?
- What type of exercise or activity can I do that I would enjoy doing?
- How can I fuel my system with the right food it requires?
- Why do I have to eat better quality foods?
- Why should I exercise today?

THE 9 KEY HABITS OF HEALTHY FOLKS

Now that you are familiar with the primary stages of phases of healing, within chiropractic, we can move on to the nine essential habits, which healthy people practice daily, that are vital for their health. This information will help you make better decisions!

These nine habits will change your lifestyle, one step at a time. It is essential to take on a gradual and slow approach when implementing major changes in your life. If you do not, you are likely to burn out and may give up, convincing yourself that the change was a bad idea or something you did not want. Here are the fundamental principles:

1. Water/Hydration

We drink coffee and soda daily but can tend to be negligent when it comes to drinking enough water. Water is vital to our health — after all, 95% of our system is composed of water, not coffee or carbonated drinks. Furthermore, water can expel toxins from our system. Various studies have confirmed that drinking at least eight glasses of water daily can substantially impact the system's power to preserve health, and fight off illness.

2. Veggies

Some people may think vegetables are unappetizing, but our parents were not wrong when they made us eat our vegetables, especially green ones, which are full of vitamins, like spinach and broccoli. Increasing your daily consumption of greens is one of the wisest nutritional choices you can make for your health. Consider this, from a scientific perspective: When plants grow, they utilize light to transform it into energy, by a procedure called "photosynthesis." You are in essence taking this energy from the plants, by consuming wholesome and raw, leafy greens.

3. Antioxidant Nutrients

Antioxidants are the key to handling the destructive "free radicals", which are oxygen-containing molecules that can cause cell damage and certain chemical reactions, such as oxidation. An excessive amount of free radicals have been connected to many forms of illness and disease, such as cancer. Free radicals are not just triggered by the natural aging process, but also by other factors such as stress, injuries, or a bad diet, rich in processed and chemical-loaded foods.

Our parents always told us to eat our veggies and fruits, and they had a good point. Green vegetables, fruits, and nuts are naturally fortified with antioxidants and nutrients.

A nutritious diet composed of powerful antioxidants makes the body more capable of fighting off and eradicating, inflammatory diseases and issues, such as heart problems, diabetes, and high blood pressure and may prevent some forms of cancer. Here's the problem, though: Only 7% of Americans eat enough antioxidant nutrients daily, even though antioxidants are readily available in fruits, vegetables, tea, and from so many other sources.

It's commonly said that the brighter the color of a fruit or vegetable is, the more antioxidants it is likely to contain. So, how many sources of antioxidants should we get, daily? It is normally recommended to eat five portions of fruits or vegetables per day, for example, one piece of fruit with your breakfast, one-two vegetables for lunch, a piece of fruit or vegetable for a midday snack, and one of either for dinner. This is an easy addition to your diet that will pay off in the long run.

4. Healthy Oils

We tend to lack essential fatty acids in our daily life, which could benefit our health. Based on studies, the average individual suffers from a lack of vital, fatty acids of about 90%. An insufficient intake of essential fatty acids is connected to problems of the heart and brain, along with many types of inflammatory disorders. Only certain fats and oils are healthy, among which are fish and flaxseed oil.

5. Proper Oxygenation

It is essential to allow for proper oxygenation of body tissues, through mindful breathing methods, which are supported by cardio exercise. In reality, very few of us ever learn how to breathe correctly!

6. A Good Posture

We cannot breathe properly if we are also dealing with a bad posture. The way we stand or sit can put a strain on how well we breathe, and a bad posture can lead to other issues. It puts stress on the spinal curve, which in turn causes problems with the nervous system.

7. Physical Activity/Exercise

We know this point can be a challenge, especially if exercise is not a part of your daily regimen, but exercise and physical activity are vital to your health. Your system needs a complete cardio workout plan that activates the vital muscles in your body, such as the heart. You have to challenge it, to have it pump more blood and oxygen throughout your body.

8. Adequate Sleep

It's no surprise that the average American lacks sufficient sleep. We are reportedly so busy that we neglect the necessity for proper sleep regularly. The issue is that insufficient sleep is a known culprit in poor health. People who don't sleep enough have a higher risk of suffering from the consequences of a poor immune system. So, besides inducing tiredness and fatigue, lack of sleep can also lead to the onset of other issues due to suppressed immunity.

9. Positive Mindset

It is possible to be "overly positive", but there is a valid point to having a positive mindset. If you catch a cold, complaining and moaning about it will only make you feel worse. However, if you approach it with a positive outlook and focus on getting better, instead of cursing it and paying attention to feeling ill, you will likely recover more quickly.

If you practice these nine lifestyle habits and incorporate them into your life, it is much more likely that you will create a healthier, happier reality for yourself.

CHAPTER 13

SPINAL DEGENERATION

Spinal degeneration refers to the spine's gradual loss of structure and function in response to mechanical or metabolic injury. Intervertebral discs, joints, ligaments, and bones may go through morphological changes that are referred to as degenerative. The spine is the central part of our body, providing structural support, shielding neural elements, and aiding in trunk movement. Spine consists of two adjacent vertebras, with the intervertebral disc, spinal ligaments, and facet joints forming a functional spinal unit. The intervertebral disc contains the nucleus pulposus centrally, the annulus fibrosus peripherally, and the cartilaginous endplates on the anterior and posterior sides at the junction of the vertebral body.

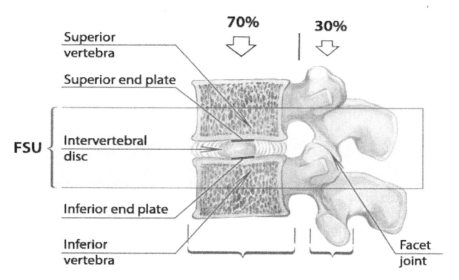

Image 1: Functional Spinal Unit. 70% of compression is distributed through intervertebral discs and the vertebral body, and the remaining 30% is through facet joints. Image Source: Kushchayev et al., 2018

The degeneration of the spine may involve other elements of FSU too, termed as horizontal or segmental degeneration, or it may lead to adjacent segment disease affecting adjacent FSU, thus changing the entire biomechanics of the spine. Spinal degeneration can be divided into three categories based on location and sequence of development.

- A. The degenerative process usually starts within the Nucleolus pulposus, a highly viscous and elastic gelatinous structure consisting of proteoglycans and intermolecular water. This degeneration causes the nucleolus pulposus to dry out, resulting in reduced intradiscal pressure.
- B. It then extends to the adjacent vertebrae's annulus fibrosus, discs, end plates, and bone marrow.

C. Further degeneration finally affects distant structures leading to facet joint osteoarthritis, hypertrophy of ligamentum flavum, and spinal canal stenosis.

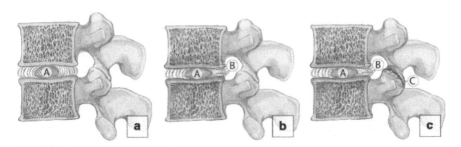

Image 2: Degenerative Changes of Spine.
Image Source: Kushchayev et al., 2018

Prevalence of Spinal degeneration

Spinal disorders represent the most common problems worldwide. Global Burden of Disease Study 2013 reported that low back pain was the foremost cause of disability, with an increase of 56.75% from 1990 to 2013. Neck problem was considered the fourth leading cause, with a 54% increase from 1990 to 2013.

Hebrew Senior Life's Institute for Aging Research and Boston Medical Center conducted the research (2018). It stated that 1/3 of people 40-59 years of age have image-based evidence of moderate to severe degenerative disease, and more than half suffer from mild to severe spinal osteoarthritis. The incidence of disc narrowing, and joint osteoarthritis has shown a 2 to 4-fold increase in those between 60-69 and 70-89, respectively. These events are found to be occurring 40 - 70% more often in women than men.

Factors Leading to Spinal degeneration/ Early degeneration

Spinal degeneration, including disc narrowing and joint osteoarthritis, leads to pain, reduced function, and increased healthcare costs. The leading causes of disc degeneration include genetics, age, insufficient nutrient supply, and mechanical loading, making the discs weaker and prone to loss of structural and functional ability during daily activities. Simply put, spinal degeneration is caused by stress and neglect.

- ❖ Aging: Spinal degeneration is common in old age. As age progresses, one has more years for things to "go bad" and also more days possible to avoid doing healthy things for their spine. But age alone is not responsible for spinal degeneration. Most spinal x-rays show different levels with varying amounts of degeneration. If age were the factor causing spinal degeneration, then all levels would equally degenerate because they are all the same age. Instead, there are varying degrees of spinal degeneration. Again, that is because spinal degeneration is caused by stress and neglect, not old age.
- ❖ Genetics: Genetics can also play an essential role in the early degeneration of the spine. Many genes are involved in the degenerative process in humans, like genes coding for collagen I, IX (COL9A2 and COL9A3), collagen XI (COL11A2), Interleukin-1, aggrecan, vitamin D receptor, matrix metalloproteinase 3, and CILP. Boyd et al. (2008)

researched a mice model to analyze the association between genetics and the early onset of disc degeneration. They reported deletion mutation in collagen IX leads to musculoskeletal degeneration of bone and cartilaginous tissue regions.

- ❖ Insufficient nutrient supply: Disc requires nutrients like oxygen and Glucose to perform its activity. Failure to achieve these nutrients causes disc cells to lose their ability to synthesize and maintain the disc extracellular matrix, eventually leading to disc degeneration. The cells depend on blood vessels to supply nutrients and remove metabolic waste. Diseased conditions like sickle cell anemia, Caisson disease, Gaucher's disease, and atherosclerosis affect the blood supply to the vertebral body and can cause disc degeneration. The frequency of long-term or no exercise also affects the supply of nutrients and their concentration in tissues. Another factor contributing to insufficient nutrient supply is the calcification of end plates where blood supply is not disturbed, but nutrients cannot reach the disc cells.
- ❖ Mechanical load/ injury: abnormal mechanical loads or injuries also lead to spinal degeneration and back pain as they cause structural damage. Heavy load, driving, and strenuous physical work are the major factors contributing to the degenerative process.
- ❖ Environmental factors: Various environmental factors are also involved in spinal degeneration.

Smoking is also found to have modest relation with disc degeneration. Oda et al. (2004) conducted the research in a rat smoking model. They found that inhalation of tobacco smoke leads to the production of inflammatory cytokines, destroying chondrocyte activity.

Treatment Of Spinal Degeneration:

The aim of treatment is to minimize pain, maintain mobility, and stabilize the spine.

Non-Surgical Treatment:

- Medications: various medications are used to relieve pain associated with disc degeneration.
- Non-steroidal anti-inflammatory drugs like ibuprofen, Naproxen & Cox 2 inhibitors to reduce pain and inflammation.
- Muscle relaxants may also sometimes be helpful and are prescribed to relieve muscle spasms
- Steroids: oral steroids such as methylprednisolone are prescribed for severe pain.
- Narcotics: codeine, hydrocodone, and oxycodone are reserved for severe pain and are used for a short period due to their addictive effect.
- Tramadol: it is a non-narcotic drug used as a pain reliever being more potent than NSAIDs
- Antiseizure Medications: they are specifically used to relieve the nerve pain caused by degeneration of discs, as in sciatica or peripheral neuropathy, i.e., Gabapentin

- ❖ Facet Joint Injections: these are used to relieve the pain of facet joints by injecting steroids and local anesthetic. The most commonly used long-acting steroids are methylprednisolone, triamcinolone, and betamethasone.
- ❖ Chiropractic Care: it is effective in reversing spinal degeneration. Multimodal spinal rehabilitation with vibration traction therapy was given to patients with herniated and bulging discs. Positive outcomes were achieved in increasing disc height, pain rating, and functional rating index.
- ❖ Massage Therapy: Massage therapy may include soft-tissue manipulation, neuromuscular techniques, fascial work, stretching, self-stretching, joint play, and hydrotherapy. Following massage therapy with cervical degeneration and neck pain, there was a significant decrease in pain and an increase in functional activities.
- ❖ Physical Therapy: patients with degenerative disc disease should undergo physical therapy before opting for surgical treatments. Upon comparing with operative treatment for patients with back pain and degenerative disc disease, no significant difference in long-term outcomes regarding health status, disability, and pain was observed
- ❖ DRX9000® True Non-Surgical Spinal Decompression®: DRX9000® therapy is an effective treatment used to help heal and regenerate injured discs. As opposed to most treatments that attempt to alter or mask the symptoms of pain, DRX9000®

therapy can help draw in bulging or herniated discs away from the nerves and also draws moisture and nutrients into the disc, which can rehydrate and thicken a degenerated disc. DRX9000® therapy is a fantastic and safe alternative to risky spinal surgeries or injections.

Surgical Treatment

- ❖ Spinal Fusion: it is the most common operative approach used today. It involves bridging two or more vertebrae using bone tissue achieved by autografts from the iliac crest or lamina. Alternative to iliac crest may be allografts, demineralized bone matrix (DBM), ceramics, and bone morphogenetic proteins. This surgical treatment aims to stabilize the movement and eradicate the degeneration of discs. Most recently, spinal fusions often include metal hardware (rods and screws) instead of or in addition to bone grafts.
- ❖ Total Disc Replacement: In this procedure, IVD is replaced. This surgical procedure is carried out to restore intervertebral discs' functionality, resist wear, relieve pain, and avoid disability and degeneration of adjacent discs and facet joints. TDR is contraindicated in lumbar spinal stenosis, chronic fractures, instability as in spondylolisthesis, Osteoporosis, and infection.
- ❖ Nucleus Replacement: this replaces the IVD nucleus while preserving endplates and annulus. This technique doesn't benefit degenerative

changes already present in end plates and annulus. Various materials and designs have been used to replace the nucleus to stabilize movement, preserve disc height and reshare load with the annulus. Most commonly used in prosthetic disc nuclei consisting of geometric cores enclosed in polyethylene.

- ❖ Stabilization: An alternative spinal fusion approach is stabilization through semi-rigid or dynamic implants. Semi-rigid stabilization helps achieve fusion without stress shielding at the bone graft that may disturb or delay bridging. Dynamic stabilization helps to stabilize by restricting painful movement without discectomy and fusion.
- ❖ Ablation Therapy: it is a minimally invasive technique using radiofrequency energy to destroy abnormal tissue around facet joints and help relieve pain. An endoscopic radiofrequency denervation is a practical approach for providing long-term pain relief from facet joints. American Society of Interventional Pain Physicians recommends percutaneous rhizotomy for relieving chronic neck and back pain originating from facet joints.

Standard Of Care To Treat Cervical Spine Conditions:

Cervical Spondylosis or degeneration causes the spinal cord and nerve root compression, which may lead to pain and disability. It is also presented by radiculopathy (pain & reduced reflexes) and myelopathy (spasticity and weakness with or without numbness).

Cervical degeneration is common with neck, shoulder, and brachial pain, which often does not require surgical treatment. Surgery is generally used to decompress the spinal cord and nerve roots.

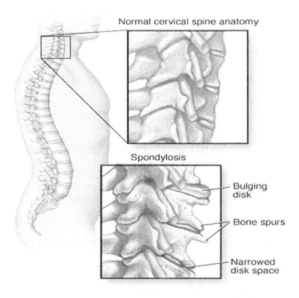

Image 3: Cervical Spine and Spondylosis.
Image Source: Scoliosis SOS Clinic, 2018

Non-Operative Treatment:

- ❖ Transforaminal epidural steroid injections, Ozone injections, cervical traction, medications, and physical therapy effectively manage pain and treat cervical degenerative disease (NASS).
- ❖ Use of ice can provide quick relief. Motion exercises to maintain movement of facet joints and posture, Resistance rehabilitation, and home exercises are also helpful.

Surgical Procedures: Surgical procedures may be anterior or posterior, depending upon the site of root compression.

- Posterior Approach: these are primarily recommended in patients with posterior cervical compression, stenosis, and lordotic cervical alignment.
- Cervical Laminectomy: it involves the removal of the lamina to relieve pressure from the spinal cord or nerve and is indicated for the management of cervical myelopathy
- Cervical Laminoplasty: an alternative to laminectomy in treating cervical myelopathy.
- Cervical laminectomy/ laminoplasty with fusion: to overcome the complications of long-term instability with laminectomy/ laminoplasty, this technique has evolved for managing cervical myelopathy.
- Cervical laminoforaminotomy: it is recommended for surgical management of radiculopathy
- Anterior Approach: it is indicated for patients with short segment stenosis and kyphotic cervical alignment.
- Anterior Cervical Interbody Fusion: the use of anterior discectomy and fusion is increasing because of less tissue damage and avoidance of spinal canal exposure.
- Cervical Disc Arthroplasty: it is used for the restoration of a failed intervertebral disc with functional disc prosthesis

Medication Treatment for Cervical Spinal Degeneration

Oral medications are the treatment of choice. These include:

- Narcotics: these are recommended for short-term treatment.
- Non-Steroidal Anti-inflammatory drugs: Aspirin, Ibuprofen, and OTC drugs are effective in pain relief. Cox 2 inhibitors are also effective.
- Corticosteroids: as dexamethasone, they are more effective in arm pain than neck pain.
- Muscle relaxants: used to relieve muscle spasms and dysesthesia.
- Anti-depressants: amitriptyline to relieve depression and neuropathic pain and improve sleep. Duloxetine is mainly recommended for relieving depression as well arthritic pain.
- Neuroleptic medications: such as gabapentin and Pregabalin. Gabapentin is prescribed for neuropathic and spinal nerve pain. Pregabalin treats fibromyalgia and is used to relieve radicular pain.
- Steroids with Anesthetic: Facet joint injections in which long-acting corticosteroid is given with long-acting anesthetic.

Surgical Procedures for Cervical Spinal Degenerative disorders

- *Radiculopathy:* Surgical procedure may be anterior or posterior depending upon the site of root compression. The anterior approach usually involves removing osteophytes above and below the disc spaces and placing a bone graft. Posterior approaches are valuable in root decompression, avoiding the need for discectomy.
- *Cervical spondylotic myelopathy:* Chronic disc degeneration with osteophytes is detected at C5/C6 and C6/C7. Surgery is carried out either by anterior or posterior approach.
- *Neck pain:* Spinal degeneration occurs at C2/C3. Cervical spinal fusion is Carried out occasionally for neck pain with cervical spondylosis but is not a suggested practice.
- *Rheumatoid Arthritis*: Atlantoaxial subluxation is the misalignment of C1/C2 cervical vertebrae and is the most common cervical indicator of rheumatoid arthritis. Such cases with myelopathy and subluxation need urgent fusion. Even with minor subluxation, patients may be referred for surgical assessment. The posterior approach is considered with the placement of screws across the C1/C2 and immediate bone grafting. This is a highly recommended method as it has improved pain and quality of life.

Outcomes of Surgical Procedures

The morbidity rate is higher in all cervical surgeries, so the benefit to risk ratio is to be determined before surgery other than chronic severe pain and progressive motor disorders. Surgery for radiculopathy has shown excellent outcomes in 90% of cases. For myelopathy, 48% showed improvement if treated within a year of symptoms, and only 16% showed improvement after a year or more. Surgical procedures are required for the rapid relief of cervical radiculopathy from degenerative disorders (NASS)

- ❖ Anterior cervical discectomy with or without fusion is a similar treatment approach in treating single-level cervical radiculopathy associated with degeneration.
- ❖ Anterior cervical discectomy with fusion and Post lateral fusion for single-level degeneration in cervical radiculopathy are considered to achieve similar outcomes.
- ❖ ACDF and total disc arthroplasty (TDA) are also considered comparable treatments with successful short-term outcomes for degenerative cervical radiculopathy

Long-Term Outcomes

Long-term outcomes for spinal surgery tend to be poor. Because spinal surgery addresses the symptoms of pain more than the degenerative process of the spine, even if one comes through the surgery with improvement in their symptoms, it is usually short-lived because the degenerative process was not addressed and will continue unabated. In surgical fusion, the degenerative process usually progresses even quicker because the everyday stress from the fused segments is redistributed to the areas above and below that fused segment. When the surrounding levels are stressed, they degenerate quickly, the patient gets symptoms of pain again, and often the surgical fusions continue to spread as the degenerative processes spread. We've all heard the saying, "There's no such thing as one back surgery."

Incidence of surgical interventions:

Most people with cervical degeneration remain asymptomatic. 10-15% of cases are referred to surgical procedures following the worst condition.

Side effects/Complications of medication treatment

Medications are considered to relieve pain in cervical degenerative disease, but they may lead to mild to severe complications. Some of the common side effects of these medications are:

- ❖ Anti-inflammatory medications: Nausea, gastric ulcers, and kidney dysfunction are commonly observed. They have an increased risk of cardiac dysfunction in patients with cardiac issues.
- ❖ Steroids: Side effects include hyperglycemia, weight gain, osteoporosis, and gastric ulcers.
- ❖ Muscle relaxants tend to be abused and lead to sedation, fatigue, and depression. They should be used for a shorter duration.

- ❖ Neuroleptic drugs: Sedation, weight gain, and depression are the common side effects.
- ❖ Opioids: Side effects include constipation, sedation, depression, dependence, and abuse. Their long-term use is not recommended as they lead to addiction.

Short term & Long-term complications after surgery

Surgeries for cervical radiculopathy and myelopathy are associated with complications that may sometimes be fatal.

- ❖ Post-operative infections have also been reported after cervical spine surgeries with an incidence rate of 0-18%. Infection is more common in the posterior approach than in the anterior one.
- ❖ Other short complications are postoperative pain, pelvic fracture, nerve palsy, and chronic donor site pain.
- ❖ Surgery is carried out to decompress the spinal cord and nerve roots, which may destabilize the cervical spine by invasion with muscles, ligaments, or bone, leading to severe neck pain either by anterior or posterior approach.
- ❖ There is a high rate of radiological kyphotic deformity of the upper back spine, shown by the outward curve after surgery at the fusion level.
- ❖ C5 Motor palsy is a frequent complication after cervical spine decompression by posterior approach.

- Other complications include esophageal perforation, carotid/vertebral artery injury, or neural structures injuries reported in 1-8% of patients.
- Death from surgery has also been reported varying from 0-1.8%.

<u>Global Burden Of Disability With Neck Pain:</u> Disability-Adjusted Life Years (DALYs) from neck pain increased from 23.9 million to 33.6 million (47%) in 1990-2010. Neck pain is reported to be the 4th leading cause of disability, with an annual prevalence of 15-50%.

<u>Revision Surgeries:</u> Revision surgeries are often required for cervical spine conditions. The rate of revision varies with the type of surgery.

- Anterior cervical decompression and fusion have a 2-year revision of 2.1-9.13% for single-level surgery and 4.4-10.7% for multilevel. The need for revision surgery is mainly due to adjacent segment disease, which has the appearance of new symptoms every year.
- Cervical disc arthroplasty has a revision rate of 1.8-5.4% at two years to 2.9% at five years.
- Posterior Procedures such as cervical foraminotomy has a revision rate of 2.9% at seven years, laminoplasty at 2.1% at 15 years, laminectomy at 2%, and fusion at 27% at 3 to 4 years.

Co-management with specialists:

Degenerative cervical spine conditions require proper management and treatment. To achieve better outcomes and long-term positive effects, expert opinion and cooperation is required from surgeons, neurologists, rheumatologists, physiatrists, rehabilitation medicine specialist, and primary care physicians. If you are looking for natural solutions, look for a Pierce Results System-certified chiropractor.

CHAPTER 14

SCOLIOSIS

The causes of scoliosis are not yet well understood, although this is a relatively common problem affecting about 5% of children and adolescents and about 2% to 3% of the total population. Scoliosis is a permanent condition of the spine which occurs when the spine is "off-center" and grows laterally, eventually turning into an "S" or a "C" shape. This condition causes a lot of uneven pressure, strain, and pain.

Unfortunately, when patients are diagnosed with scoliosis, they are told it is "idiopathic." This means that the development of the condition, or the cause, is sudden and not fully known. It also infers that treatment will be difficult, with uncertain outcomes.

For decades, scoliosis has been considered a difficult and somewhat mysterious condition. Although there is no definitive cure, the best way to alleviate symptoms and prevent a further progression of the condition would be to resolve its underlying cause. A traditional treatment approach is based on support techniques, the prescription of anti-inflammatory drugs, and spinal surgery. These *can* offer relief of symptoms but are not without risk and do not handle the condition's root cause.

Some people who undergo chiropractic adjustments and back exercises may see 10 – 30% improvements in just a few months. Although this is not a complete cure, it can stop the progression of the deformation of the spinal curvature and thus help avoid unnecessary or irreversible surgeries.

Signs and Symptoms of Scoliosis

Symptoms usually begin to develop during adolescence, especially at puberty. However, older adults with back pain may also be diagnosed with scoliosis at a late age.

What is Scoliosis? Here are some common signs and symptoms:

- Back pain (up to 90% of patients with scoliosis reported back pain).
- The body tilts or slants to one side.
- One shoulder blade appears to be larger than the other.
- One hip appears to be placed higher up than the other
- The head is not carried at a line directly above the pelvis or midline.
- The spine appears to develop, laterally, into an "S" or a "C" shape (studies show that the S-shaped curvature is more likely to worsen than the C-

shaped curvature. Curvature development in the mid-thoracic spine becomes more severe than in the upper or lower part of the spine.)
- Tingling or acute numbness in the extremities, fingers, or toes.
- A loss of balance.
- Accelerated aging of the intervertebral discs.
- Decreased lung capacity.

Scoliosis Data: Prevalence, Risk Factors, and Complications

- Scoliosis is a problem that also affects school children, with the primary age of onset and diagnosis being between 10 to 15 years.
- Reports show that about 80% of patients with scoliosis receive an idiopathic diagnosis. This leaves many patients and their families with a sense of insecurity and frustration about the outcome, although there is hope that natural treatments can have a significant, positive impact.
- The exact causes of scoliosis are unknown, but contributing factors are congenital malformations, such as "congenital scoliosis" (a type of hereditary scoliosis), spinal cord injuries, and issues with the muscles and nerves, like muscular dystrophy.
- Many patients and their families are often offered one of three treatment options: 1) "Watch and Wait," where the patient is asked to "wait" and "watch" for six months and come back for a reassessment to see if the condition has worsened. 2)

Apply the treatment with orthotics (wearing braces or splints). 3) Undergo spinal surgery, such as bone removal and removal of vertebrae or implants of metal plates, as some of the more common options.
- Each year, scoliosis patients make more than 600,000 visits to private medical practices. An estimated 30,000 children undergo vertebral body tethering, or "VBT" (a surgery where a strong chord, a "tether," is attached to the spine to help the spine grow into a more normal shape). In contrast, 38,000 patients undergo spinal fusion surgery.
- Complications can occur when muscles and body tissues deform over time as the body tries to compensate for the abnormal torsion and flexion of the spine. These complications may continue to develop even after spinal surgery.
- During a "Watch and Wait" period, many cases continue to worsen while they could receive care. With cases that wait further, studies have reported an average increase of 2.4 degrees per year over five years. Moreover, among adolescents, scoliosis has increased by more than 10 degrees, on average, after age 22.
- Besides posture, scoliosis can also affect the quality of life as it can cause pain, interfere with normal lung function, and impair sleep and the ability to exercise and live normally. A poor body image is also common; repeated X-rays can increase the risk of severe radiation exposure problems.

How Does Scoliosis Develop?

Scoliosis is essentially a symptom of a deeper biological problem. It causes a mechanical spine malfunction, although the degree to which this happens and how it affects spinal curvature and alignment varies from patient to patient. Although scoliosis treatment approaches work best when they are personalized, and the unique history of the patient has been taken into account, several things work well for most patients:

- Improving the diet
- Receiving chiropractic care
- Practicing specific spinal exercises

Patients with scoliosis may experience various symptoms and degrees of severity, depending on the progression of their condition. No one patient suffers the same degree of damage, bone density, deformation, or spine curvature. Many people develop some degree of abnormal spinal alignment, but this is usually not diagnosed unless the curvature of the spine rotates at an angle of 10 degrees or more. At this point, it is then classified as "true scoliosis."

In some cases, what starts as a small deformation in the curvature of the spine tends to worsen over time. Especially if the curvature of the spine twists in the middle, this causes the ribcage to disengage from its normal position. If someone incurs a vortex curvature of more than 30 degrees, the condition is more likely to progress in severity. A 60-degree curvature can lead to many complications, including breathing difficulties.

On average, people with scoliosis suffer a reduction in life expectancy of up to 14 years due to the stress on the heart and the decreased supply of oxygen to the body. Scoliosis is also associated with headaches, difficulty breathing, digestive problems, chronic diseases, and pain in the hip, knees, and legs.

The Underlying Causes of Scoliosis

Patients with scoliosis can come from all walks of life. Children and middle-aged older people; can all develop this condition. However, the condition seems to affect women more than men. While both sexes can develop scoliosis, estimates show that two to three times more women develop the disease than men.

Mild cases of scoliosis are prevalent in the general population, but not everyone's noticeably affected. The risk of developing any form of scoliosis increases with age, and research shows that patients are diagnosed mainly at 10-15 years old. It also affects 3 - 5% of adolescents and usually occurs in the prepubertal years. Furthermore, recent studies have shown that the prevalence of scoliosis in the elderly can reach up to 68%.

The exact cause of scoliosis is not known or commonly agreed upon. Still, it seems to be due to a combination of genetic factors, lifestyle, and environmental factors, such as:

- The nutrition of a patient
- Family history
- Abnormal bone development
- Hormonal imbalances
- Possible problems in the areas of the brain that monitors adequate symmetry in bone growth, spinal alignment, or balance

Risk Factors For Scoliosis: Who Suffers The Most?

Although some aspects of the condition are still considered mysterious, it is a known factor that patients with scoliosis often have several things in common:

- An unbalanced diet (especially regarding magnesium, vitamin D, and vitamin K deficiencies)
- Hypermobility, such as "double joint" or "chest depression," PE (Pectus Excavatum)
- A poor posture
- Delayed development in puberty and other hormonal problems in adolescents (a condition of estrogen deficiency or hypoestrogenism)
- Women who are postmenopausal or hypoestrogenic have an increased risk of developing scoliosis, as estrogen plays an essential role in the formation of bone density
- Athletes with low body weight, poor bone health, or who incur nutritional deficiencies are similarly at risk

- Individuals who suffer from other conditions that may co-occur with scoliosis, including connective tissue disease, sciatic nerve pain, mitral valve prolapse (a problem with valvular heart disease, where the damage takes place in any of the four heart valves), Down's syndrome, osteoporosis, and osteopenia
- Genetic predispositions which affect the bones and health of the spine (scoliosis runs in the family line, and some mutated genes appear to increase the risk of hereditary forms of scoliosis)

Some people assume that genetic factors are the primary or only reason for the development of scoliosis. Research has shown, though, that scoliosis recurs between family members 25% - 35% of the time. This is believed to be due to specific genetic mutations that affect how our bones use and store calcium. Nevertheless, genes are not considered the sole cause of this condition.

Regarding a predisposition to scoliosis, it is essential to remember that our genes are not our destiny. We can do many things to compensate for hereditary factors that make us more susceptible to disease development, including scoliosis. For example, a healthy diet can significantly help to balance our nutritional content (including calcium and magnesium) and help switch specific genes on or off, which affect our growth and development.

Now that you understand what contributes to the development of scoliosis, it will help you clarify some myths about the disease. It is a common misconception that carrying heavy objects, sleeping in certain positions, or suffering injury can cause scoliosis, but facts do not support this. These daily activities can lead to poor posture and cause other back problems, but they are not the leading cause of scoliosis.

Diagnosis of Scoliosis

Historically, schools have made children perform the "Adam's Forward Bend Test, "which allows a doctor or school nurse to evaluate the curvature of their spine and detect abnormalities in the ribcage. This is still done today, but recently it has been shown that these tests are not necessarily accurate and miss diagnosing some cases of scoliosis. For this reason, this test is not the most reliable form of screening children for scoliosis, especially not those coming from families with a known medical history of the disease.

The ScoliScore AIS Prognostic Test is a genetic test that can predict the likelihood of a child developing scoliosis. It is a saliva test currently used to study the genes that may affect the development of the spine and indicate the possibility of a young person developing severe abnormalities. It is believed to be a very accurate test (about 99%) and can predict whether a slight curvature of the spine will progress and develop into a severe curvature or deformity.

As this test can predict scoliosis early on, it can help prevent patients from future surgery or unnecessary medication.

Suppose you suspect that you or your child have scoliosis. In that case, your physician may perform X-rays to measure the spine's curvature, observe the angle of the various vertebrae, and assess whether or not the spine twists unevenly to one side. Physicians can diagnose cases of scoliosis using "the Cobb angle." This can quantify the degree of sideways curvature of the spine and help determine the progression of any deformation.

Treating Scoliosis Naturally

Over time the "Watch and Wait" approach, strengthening the spinal musculature, and performing corrective spinal surgery have not always been practical and are risky approaches. However, chiropractic or osteopathic manipulation therapy, in combination with deep massage and physiotherapy to strengthen the core, can have significant and positive results.

Scoliosis has no known cure but can be controlled and managed more naturally than drugs and surgery. Similar to other chronic conditions, such as diabetes and high blood pressure, it has been discovered that the faster a scoliosis patient can begin natural management of the condition, the better their results will be. However, there are some notable issues regarding the most traditional and common treatment options:

- A 2007 study found that 23% of orthopedic patients still ended up undergoing spinal fusion surgery, despite treatment, compared to 22% of patients who did nothing.

- Orthoses generally cause emotional scarring, especially in children and adolescents, who experience a negative body image, pain, skin abrasions, and issues with bone growth. One study found that 60% of patients treated with an orthosis could become dependent on it, and 14% thought the experience left a psychological scar.
- Whether support for the spine can halt the developing deformation, benefits can be lost once the orthosis is removed and surgery is still needed.
- Spinal surgery carries a high risk of permanent paralysis, infection, and other severe health issues.

Lifestyle Changes and Chiropractic Care May Help Treat Scoliosis

An article from 2004, "Treatment of Scoliosis by a Combination of Manipulative Therapy and Rehabilitation: A Retrospective Case Series," was published by Drs. Morningstar, Woggon, and Lawrence at BMC Musculoskeletal Disorders have changed how we view scoliosis treatments and chiropractic care. Other studies have supported chiropractic and orthopedic care, equipment, and treatment.

These methods also present a lower risk of causing permanent damage and severe side effects and allow the patients to manage their conditions. In terms of care, the medical costs are also less than conventional treatments and much less invasive than corrective surgery.

Dr. Eric Jaszewski was the lead author of original scoliosis research from 2016 in the Journal of Pediatric, Maternal, and Family Health – Chiropractic.

It was entitled: "Improvement in Idiopathic Scoliotic and Sub-Scoliotic Curvatures Following Subluxation Correction Utilizing the Pierce Results System: A Retrospective Analysis of Outcomes" and was co-authored by: Jessica Harden, DC, and Mark Smith, DC.

This study intended to demonstrate the effectiveness of the Pierce Results System of vertebral subluxation analysis and correction in 14 patients with adolescent idiopathic scoliosis and 22 patients with 'sub-scoliotic' spinal curvatures. It demonstrates a group trend towards structural change within the scoliosis subgroup of 25.96% over an average of 4.75 specific spinal adjustments. An even more significant trend towards correction of 51.84% over an average of 6.41 adjustments was found in the sub-scoliosis group who started care with curvatures of 7-10 degrees. Six subjects in this group experienced 100% correction at their first re-examination x-ray.

This was, at the time, the second most extensive study to date to objectively examine the results of a group of patients with adolescent idiopathic scoliosis from a random sampling in an individual practice following a treatment protocol involving specific spinal adjustment alone.

Dr. Eric was also a co-author of the follow-up study in 2017 in the same journal: "Reduction and Maintenance of Scoliotic and Sub-Scoliotic Curvatures: A Follow-Up Study on Children with Idiopathic Scoliosis Undergoing Subluxation Correction with Pierce Results System."

- — 20 of the original 36 subjects were included in a follow-up study.
- — Scoliosis – 14.4% initially, additional 7.6%
- — Sub-group – 61.5% initially, additional 18.2%
- — Total reduction – 46.8%

This is the first retrospective case series to follow up on chiropractic management of idiopathic scoliosis. During chiropractic care, which ranged anywhere from one to four years, a continual trend of structural improvement was observed.

These facts make the Pierce Results System, specifically Dr. Eric Jaszewski, uniquely qualified to apply modern, effective, non-surgical, non-invasive chiropractic care to assist patients suffering from scoliosis.

CHAPTER 15

TEXT NECK

You've probably been told once or twice to stop constantly looking at your phone. Using it is almost unavoidable though, since smartphones are such multi-functional devices and a big part of our lives. Unfortunately, it turns out that the convenience of being able to reply to emails, send text messages, and take calls on your smartphone might be taking a toll on your body.

So What Is "Text Neck"?

Text neck is a term that refers to the bent-neck position assumed when people look at their phones. It is being warned against by spinal surgeons who have noticed an increase in the number of patients with neck and upper-back pain (likely due to prolonged smartphone use), according to Reuters Health. Text neck is being described as a modern ailment that is due to spending long periods staring down at your mobile phone, tablet, or other devices.

Usually, when you respond to a message or scroll through an app, you pull out your phone and look down at it. It's not uncommon (albeit slightly jarring) to see a group of people together with everyone's heads bent down, staring at their respective phones.

Recent research shows that smartphone users are spending an average of four hours each day staring at their device (that's 1,400 hours each year!). Because of this, it is no wonder that the incidence of 'text neck' is on the rise. It seems that this relatively new phenomenon is becoming more common with the increasing prevalence of mobile technology, particularly among younger generations.

What Causes Text Neck?

Does anyone not have a smartphone these days? Using a smartphone all the time can actually impact your posture, and most people don't even realize it! Text neck happens when you use your neck, back, and shoulder muscles too much by staying in a hunched-over position; this is usually the position you're in when you spend a lot of time looking down and forward, like when you're looking at your phone or tablet.

Text neck is an overuse syndrome or a repetitive stress injury to the neck, caused by holding your head in a forward and downward position for extended periods of time. When holding your head in this position, excessive amounts of tension are created in the deep muscles of your neck and across the shoulders, causing both acute and chronic neck pain. Chronic headaches have also been linked to this condition.

The average head weighs around 11 to 14 lbs., and the cervical spine (your neck) is designed so that it will balance the weight of the head effortlessly. It even has a slight backward curve to absorb the shocks and impacts of moving around. However, as we bend our heads forward, the amount of stress and strain on the neck increases. At a 15-degree angle, this weight is about 27 lbs.; at 30 degrees, it's 40 lbs.; and at 60 degrees, it's 60 lbs.! That is the same as having an 8-year-old child hanging unsupported off your neck for several hours each day!

When you keep yourself in this position, it can cause serious strain on the spine. Text neck is more than just a scary story that parents can tell their kids to keep them off their phones; it's a real issue that can cause pain and discomfort, and even long-term damage to your health.

What Are The Symptoms of Text Neck?

Over time, this can lead to muscle strain, pinched nerves, and herniated discs. But the most obvious immediate effect is on our posture. Just have a look around: Everyone has their head down! Poor posture can cause other problems in other organs as well. Experts say that it can reduce lung capacity by as much as 30%. It has also been linked to headaches and neurological issues, depression, and heart disease.

Stretching your body's tissues for extended periods can cause it to become sore and inflamed. Repeated stress on the vertebrae can also lead to herniated discs, pinched nerves, and eventually improper curvature of the spine. Text neck usually causes neck pain and soreness. The pain can be localized to one spot or may be diffused over an area, usually at the lower part of the neck. It can be described as a dull ache or a sharp, stabbing pain in extreme cases.

In addition, looking down at your cell phone for prolonged periods can lead to:

- Stiff Neck: Soreness and difficulty in moving the neck are usually felt when you try to move it.
- Radiating Pain: There can also be a radiation of pain into the shoulders and arms.
- Muscular Weakness: The shoulders muscles, namely the trapezius, rhomboids, and shoulder external rotators become weak
- Headache: Sub-occipital muscle tightness can lead to tension-type headaches.

Other symptoms of text neck are:

— Upper back pain ranging from a chronic, nagging pain to sharp, severe upper back muscle spasms.
— Shoulder pain and tightness that can possibly result in painful shoulder muscle spasms.
— If a cervical nerve becomes pinched, pain and neurological symptoms can radiate down your arms and into your hands (known as cervical radiculopathy).

— Text neck may also lead to chronic problems due to early onset of arthritis in the neck.

What are the long-term complications of using our phones in relation to our spine and overall health? Let's first put the situation into perspective. Mobile device usage has increased significantly and will continue to do so into the future. According to text-neck.com, Americans spend approximately two hours and forty-two minutes per day communicating and socializing on their phones. They spend even more time looking down at their mobile devices for web searching and other uses. Aside from text neck, prolonged use of mobile phones in this position can cause the following long-term complications:

<u>Increases Risk Of Chronic Pain</u>: Cell phones require constant use of your hands, especially when sending text messages and emails. Responding to messages at a rapid speed can cause pain and inflammation in the joints of the hands. Back pain is also common with increased cell phone use, especially if you hold the phone between your neck and shoulders as you multitask. Long periods of cell phone use cause you to arch your neck and hold your body in a strange posture, which can all lead to back pain.

<u>Increases Risk Of Eye Vision Problems</u>: Staring at your mobile device can cause problems with your vision later in life. Screens on mobile devices tend to be smaller than computer screens, which means you are more likely to squint and strain your eyes while reading messages. According to The Vision Council, more than 70% of

Americans are not aware (or are in denial) of the fact that they are susceptible to "digital eye strain".

<u>Radiation</u>: While it is not clear if the radiation from cellphones and other connected devices causes health issues, a group of 200 biological and health scientists from around the world are trying to raise public awareness on this issue. They are calling on the United Nations, World Health Organization, and national governments to develop strict regulations concerning cellphones that create electromagnetic fields.

It Can Trigger "Nomophobia", Or The Fear Of Being Without Your Phone: Do you know that feeling of safety you get from having a fully charged phone in your hand? Nomophobia is the opposite. It can lead you to think — often irrationally — that you are not safe without a phone in your hand.

<u>Wrist Problems</u>: Another problem that comes with overuse of smartphones is problems with the wrists. The way we hold smartphones for long durations strains them, and people usually hold their phones using the last three fingers of the hand, and their thumb, while using the forefinger to perform actions on the smartphone screen. Retaining this position for long durations, daily, tends to create pains in the wrists.

It is better to keep changing the position of the hands when holding a phone or performing other tasks, such as reading. You can put down the smartphone while lying on the bed or place it on the table when sitting, in order to look down at it instead of always holding it in your hands.

What Are Some Long-Term Complications of Text Neck?

Constantly checking our phones has become second nature to us, but this wreaks havoc on our spines and may cause our shoulders to ache and necks to stiffen up.

The posture we adapt as we stare at our phones increases the stress put on the neck, and causes excessive wear and tear that could lead to permanent damage. The problem is, in order to look at your screen, you need to bend your head forwards into a flexed or extended forward-facing position. This unnatural position actually reverses the normal backward curve of the cervical spine (your neck), and this change can be observed factually on X-rays, where a straightening or even a reversal of the normal curve of the cervical spine has been observed.

When looking down, you push your head forward, which shifts your center of gravity. This is also called Forward Head Posture (FHP) and causes your head to become heavier for your spine to carry, and puts increased pressure on your spine, neck, and back. This modern phenomenon has become common due to hand-held devices being the leading way of communicating and organizing our lives.

According to statistics, the average person spends about 90 minutes a day staring at a smart device. This may not seem long, but, added up, the average person can spend a total of 23 days per year, or 3.9 years in a lifetime, looking down at their phone. This amount of time spent looking down and slouching is enough to cause a lifetime of future problems!

You probably use your smartphone, tablet, or other electronic device more than you realize. What would be your guess as to how many times you look at it a day to check messages? A conservative estimate could maybe be 40 or 50 times per day, right? The truth is that if you double that number, you are probably still a little lower than the actual amount of times you check your phone per day. This is according to research done by British psychologists which also revealed that young adults generally use their phones approximately five hours a day - one third of the entire time they are awake!

The study also leads to the conclusion that using our phones and tablets sometimes comes out of habit, rather than an actual necessity. Dr. House, a British psychologist, agrees that there is a significant lack of awareness when it comes to technology. A study asked 23 students about how much time they think they spend on using their phones, and an app was installed on their phones to keep track of this amount. Their findings showed there was no correlation between their estimated usage and the actual phone usage. The students in this study checked their phones - on average - 85 times a day. Their estimate? Less than half of that number!

Text Neck Treatment

Our relationship with iPhones, iPads, smartphones, mobile texting devices, and Internet browsing can wreak havoc with our health. If you have ever experienced pain, tension, "pins and needles" or stiffness in your wrists, arms, shoulders, and neck, then it may be time to take action and rethink your relationship with your devices.

If left untreated, "text neck" can lead to inflammation of the neck ligaments, nerve irritation, and increased curvature of the spine. The good news is that you can take measures to prevent or lessen most forms of neck pain episodes. An early diagnosis and treatment is the easiest way to recover quickly from neck pain and to prevent any recurrence.

Text neck is conservatively managed by your physiotherapist. The main goals of treatment are to reduce the tension in your neck muscles, lower the pressure in your neck, and fix the position which makes your symptoms worse.

After your physiotherapist has assessed your lifestyle, posture, and neck, they will confirm the main issues causing your neck pain. They will utilize a range of treatments, including:

- Joint mobilizations
- Posture correction exercises
- Neck stabilization exercises
- Taping techniques
- Soft tissue massage
- Education
- Acupuncture

Management and Prevention of Text Neck

While it is nearly impossible to avoid the technologies that cause these issues, individuals can make an effort to look at their phones with a neutral spine position, and to avoid spending long hours each day in a hunched position. The good news is that the mentioned symptoms can be avoided by implementing the following:

Lifting the device: By lifting the device to your eye level, you will avoid having to tilt your head forward.

Be conscious of your online-time: By being aware of the time you spend looking at your device, you will know when it is time to "log out"! There is technology which can assist you with this, such as mobile applications like OFFTIME. These applications can monitor the amount of time you spend on your device and what apps you spend time on too. Some even alert you as to when to switch off the phone and take a breather!

Sit down when using a device: When you're walking or texting while walking, you're not only at risk of accidents, but your body will also naturally tend to look downward. If you sit down while texting, you can consciously remind yourself to lift the phone while using it, and are not in danger of other factors happening in your environment.

Don't slouch: By standing up straight with your shoulders pulled back, you will keep your body aligned to a neutral position, lessening the stress put on your back, shoulders, and neck.

Stretching regularly: Stretching exercises, like yoga and Pilates, strengthen your core and may ease muscle pain. Light stretching throughout the day can also do the trick!

Stay active: By exercising your muscles and keeping them strong, you will allow them to be better able to handle the extra stress.

Still, the main point is in reducing the amount of time we spend staring at our phones. You can't live a life through your phone, and there is a beautiful world right in front of your eyes. Just look up from time to time!

See a professional: If the symptoms persist or worsen, it's a good idea to see a chiropractor who will be able to assist you and give expert advice.

Visiting A Chiropractor For Help

Text neck is a serious issue, and one of the first things you can do to start combating its symptoms is to improve your posture. Work on keeping your back straight, your shoulders back, and try to maintain a neutral spine when using any device. This applies not only to mobile devices but also to e-readers, tablets, laptops, and computers.

Remember that when your chiropractor diagnoses you with a text neck, it may not be easy to restore the curve in your neck and get you pain-free. The damage possibly comes from hundreds of hours of keeping your head in a certain position. Nevertheless, if you are willing to give time to visit your chiropractor, you can easily treat your neck and live pain-free.

CHAPTER 16

PERFECT POSTURE

We've practiced this ever since we were kids, where we often got reprimanded for not having it and when it's used in military and exercise programs, it is essential. Yet, most of us still struggle to maintain it or do it right. What am I talking about here? Well, it's having a perfect posture.

Having a wrong or bad posture can lead to all sorts of problems with the body. Appearance-wise a bad posture can make us look unappealing; our shoulders slump and look rounded, resulting in hunchbacks and making us look sloppy.

Yet we focus a lot more on the physical appeal, without putting too much attention on the negative side effects of having poor posture. One of the biggest risks of a bad posture is long-term damage to the spine, which is the network and pathway of the body, where signals are sent back and forth from our nervous system and to the brain. A bad posture can also be a very debilitating factor to our muscles.

So, what makes an ideal posture? Athletic performance-boosting expert, Dax Moy from the UK, affirms that a bad posture is one of the key factors which contribute to bad health among some of the most developed countries. He explains that when the human frame is out of proportion, this results in poor posture and eventually imposes an unbalanced weight load on the body's vital organs and systems.

What Is Posture?

Before we talk about better posture, let us first look at what posture is. If we go back to the basics, our posture is how we carry our physique, unconsciously (without constantly thinking about it or controlling it). Our posture is linked to how our brain reacts to its surroundings and how it levels out and balances the body against the effect of gravity.

Physical Therapist Frank D'Ambrosio also states that an ideal posture means that *no* area of your spine or organs is unnecessarily squished when you stand or sit. Every time we stand, walk, sit, kneel or bend the movement we make is essentially working against the effect of gravity. Gravity, in turn, places a full and constant strain on our muscles, ligaments, and joints. An ideal posture equals a good distribution of the force of gravity's pull, evening out the pressure and strains worked on the body by the effect of its weight working against gravity.

Mr. Ambrosio has a perfect definition of what good posture is: he states that an architect uses the same gravity laws when he crafts a new house or designs a building. Similar to a home, or building with bad groundwork, a human body with a bad posture is weakened and less tolerant of the pains and problems we tend to experience later in life, due to regular wear and tear.

Dax Moy further elaborates on the fact that poor posture is the leading culprit behind arthritis, back strains, problems with the eyes, digestive issues, endocrine disturbances, feelings of anxiety, fatigue, headaches, dizziness, and period pains, to name a few. As you can see the problems and risks which arise can be many if you struggle with a poor posture.

A bad posture isn't only equal to just body pain; it can also affect your mood and your emotions. Imagine someone who is depressed, and anxious, and what that person's body posture is: Do their shoulders and head pop up confidently, carrying themselves with pride? Or do they look the exact opposite? Most of the time, they have a shrunken, slumped-over posture which is not only caused by their emotional state but the bad posture itself is affecting their mood, making the condition worse.

If you're wondering whether this might be the case or not, try this little experiment for yourself to test this out. Stand up, tall, and picture or think of something that you like, which makes you feel optimistic and enthusiastic. As you are doing this, now drop your shoulders, look down and start to breathe in a shallow manner. Do you still feel in the same pleasant mood as before? Probably not!

Here is what happens: our brain stores a majority of the physical control mechanisms and our engrained, emotional reactions to certain situations. Our feelings and emotions are specifically stored in the part of our brain called "the limbic system" (or the emotional brain), which is found in the cerebrum. Doctor R. Joseph, in his report "Catatonia", reports patients with several small wounds in their cerebrum. He explains that these people are in a catatonic status and suffer from apathy (a partial or complete lack of feelings), with slow responses to external stimuli.

He adds that lesions in this region may disengage fiber passageways, which allow emotional and motivational experiences to occur in the limbic system, causing them to become unified and illustrated by the frontal neocortex.

In simple, non-scientific words; Dr. Joseph also supports the notion that the limbic system is affected by motor regulations as well. So, based on this realization, how we carry our bodies has a clear impact on our emotional brain (the limbic system), or, said more clearly, how we feel.

Posture And Its Connection To Breathing

Based on research findings, a poor posture can be incredibly destructive to healthy and essential breathing patterns, which is very common. If your posture is misaligned, even a bit, it can affect your ease of breathing as it interferes with the functions of the diaphragm.

The diaphragm is responsible for extending our lungs so that we can receive the largest amount of air and oxygen into our lungs. When the diaphragm extends, it lets the lungs and the chest cavity enlarge so that the air is inhaled, and oxygen can be received, and distributed into the body. When the diaphragm relaxes, the lungs and chest relax too and expel "used air", put layman's terms, readying themselves for another inhalation.

Did you know that, on average, we breathe about 25,000 times a day? If your diaphragm is blocked (as a result of a bad posture), you won't be able to breathe deeply, in the manner which you should be able to. This of course results in your cells getting a lesser amount of oxygen, and they can't function at their best which can also lead to other health problems. Thus, a great posture translates to a well-functioning diaphragm and ultimately better functioning cells.

Posture And Its Connection To Headaches

Several studies demonstrate a clear link between bad posture and headaches, or neck issues. The US Cervicogenic Society considers the vast majority of headaches (70-80%) to be cervicogenic in nature. In more simple words, headaches often are linked to the scalp and neck, along with a particular nerve called the "trigeminal nerve". While some headaches are associated with trauma (from a car crash, or an accident), there also seems to be a clear connection between bad posture and cervicogenic headaches. This is because, with a normal posture, the spine grounds the head like a pillar. However, when the head is tilted forward, as with a person who slouches their head too far out from the body's center line (which means an added weight of 10-12 pounds on the neck, on average) it puts an excessive amount of stress on the upper spine.

Imagine an orange alongside a pillar, to get an idea of what we are talking about here. The difference here is that, with the heavy head hanging out in front of the pillar, this places *heavy* stress on the spinal ligaments and muscles which can lead to muscle spasms. If this goes on for an extended period, this will interfere with normal blood circulation through the spinal muscles.

If you neglect this, the muscle tissue will eventually deteriorate and die off which is a pathological condition called "necrosis". Once this tissue dies, it's replaced by weaker scar tissue, which can lead to trouble moving and pain.

Determining What Good Posture Is

The issue with determining exactly what good posture is, relates to the fact that there seems to be much controversy and opinion on what exactly constitutes "good posture". Some of us are familiar with the reprimand of "standing up straight!", but standing stiff and upright isn't actually what natural, good posture is. The spine has a natural curvature in its ideal condition, which is similar to the shape of a soft S when viewed from the side. A straight line, like a ruler, is not a good posture.

One thing which most doctors, chiropractors, and physical therapists are unanimous about: we should balance our bodies, from front to back, right to left, in perfect symmetry, and that the amount of weight and strain placed on our necks should be equally distributed. But, from a chiropractic point of view, the rejuvenation of the spinal curves is also vital. This is a newer aspect of chiropractic science, called "chiropractic biophysics". If you are looking for chiropractic care, it is vital that your physician knows about this and is aware of the importance of restoring spinal curves, apart from aligning the spinal cord itself.

Even with such chiropractic biophysics methods, a chiropractor can't fully re-align the patient's back to its original condition and some patients may require a treatment regimen with decompression techniques. The level of scarring of the ligaments along the spinal column greatly determines the progress of the patient. Additionally, other factors come into play, such as age and lifestyle habits.

Checking For The Ideal Posture

As specified earlier, the key here is perfect alignment and symmetry, when viewing the spinal cord from left to right, front to back. To assess your posture, start with your head, and check for any type of rotation or bending, which leans towards your right or left side. Then check the angle of your hips to see if one side is twisted more forward, or backward. Then check the position of your feet, when resting. Are they bending inwards or outwards slightly? If they bend to one side more than another, this will inflict a great level of stress on the skeletal system and spine.

On some occasions, our feet can reveal if there is a problem with an imbalanced spine and a bad posture.

Dax Moy also suggests other tips you can use, to improve your posture but make sure you consult your physical therapist or chiropractor first, before trying these to ensure that they don't negatively affect your treatment.

- Raise your scope of motion through various exercises which enhance flexibility, and do stretches for tight muscles.
- Perform balance exercises to assist your joints in their new structure. Pilates, Yoga, Alexander Technique, Tai Chi, and similar exercise programs are good for this purpose.
- Perform strengthening exercises in your exercise schedule, preferably those which engage the muscles in your back (again consult with your chiropractor, physician, or physical therapist for this).
- Adopt functional exercises into your workouts; exercises and movements where you have to stand tall, push, pull, twist, or rotate will help keep your body balanced and stabilized. No need to use any machines.
- Don't think that by investing only a few minutes every day that you will immediately see progress. If you adopt the wrong posture during the rest of the time, you aren't helping yourself make any progress.

CHAPTER 17

THE BENEFITS OF PRENATAL CHIROPRACTIC

The start of a new life is an opportunity to give your unborn child the very best care. These first formative months can help set the tone to which this child enters the world and grows up in it. Just as it is natural to want the very best care for the child, so it should be equally important to get the best care for the mother. Holistic care, which includes chiropractic care, provides a great number of benefits for prenatal care with few risks of any side effects.

Prenatal chiropractic adjustments are one of the best things a pregnant person can do for themselves and their baby, during pregnancy. A balanced spine and pelvis optimize the health of the mother and developing baby, as well as create conditions favoring a positive birth outcome. Pregnant women under chiropractic care frequently report shorter and easier births with fewer complications. Traditional chiropractic adjustments correct misalignments (subluxations) in the spine, which disrupts the proper performance of the nervous system and the body's controls of various muscles and organs.

No harmful side effects are known from pursuing chiropractic care throughout pregnancy. The benefits of prenatal chiropractic care are, however, plentiful. These benefits include:

Establish A Pelvic Balance: A misalignment of the pelvis is a common issue. A misaligned spine can result in a protruding abdomen, increased spinal curvature, pelvic changes, and posture changes. Any misalignment of the pelvic region can cause significant pain during pregnancy and a twist in the pelvic region can cause the muscles inside the pelvic girdle to tighten, which can cause the fetus to turn in an undesirable position. This could potentially lead to a breeched birth. Chiropractic adjustments can help to open up this cramped position, so the fetus has room to move into a more comfortable position.

Relieve Back Pain: When your body makes postural changes caused by the shift in your center of gravity, back pain is a common side effect. This is probably the reason you're considering prenatal chiropractic care in the first place! The pelvic balance achieved by chiropractic adjustments is key in relieving back pain felt during pregnancy.

Experience An Easier Labor And Delivery: Chiropractic adjustments can help shorten the time of labor and make the birthing process easier. If the mother's spine and hips are in proper alignment and all the nerves to the muscles and organs in her body are free and healthy, then the birthing can progress more easily. A healthy condition of the spine can shorten labor time, too, compared to a woman who's suffering a misalignment of the spine. A balanced pelvis allows your baby to get into the best position possible when you go into labor, and this lowers the risks of any breeched or posterior positions that could require major interventions, such as a C-section. In this way, prenatal chiropractic care eases the labor and delivery process and increases your chances of a natural, non-invasive birth.

<u>Easing of Symptoms Experienced During Pregnancy</u>: Chiropractic can help relieve uncomfortable symptoms, such as nausea or vomiting. It does not work for all women, but chiropractic is one way to try to get some relief from morning sickness. If nausea and vomiting are due in part to nerves pinched by out-of-place vertebra, an adjustment can help remedy the problem.

How Is It Different Than Other Prenatal Options?

This type of care is growing in popularity among pregnant women, as a safe alternative to taking over-the-counter painkillers or other options offered for prenatal discomfort. The International Chiropractic Pediatric Association wholeheartedly recommends prenatal chiropractic care.

The most significant difference between typical alignments and those for pregnant women, is the focus of pressure away from the abdomen. Your doctor will avoid any harmful movement or stretches that could be unsafe for the developing baby, or could cause pain to the sensitive areas following pregnancy. Much of the appointment may also be focused on the pelvic region as this area experiences a lot of stress when your body changes and adapts, in order to carry the baby.

A popular reason for choosing prenatal chiropractic care, during pregnancy is its ability to aid with the fetal positioning of the baby. This is achieved by a specific chiropractic analysis and adjustment technique, called the Webster Technique, which was developed by the late Larry Webster D.C. Webster was the founder of the International Chiropractic Pediatric Association.

By using this technique, a chiropractor can create balance in the pregnant woman's pelvis, and reduce the stress to her uterus and supporting ligaments. This balanced state has been shown to promote an ideal fetal positioning, thus decreasing the chances of a breached position of the baby at birth.

When applying chiropractic care to pregnant women, the goal is to improve overall movement and to eliminate any existing pains, especially in the lower back or pelvic areas. Using chiropractic care during pregnancy is an excellent option, as treatments are entirely natural and non-invasive. Many medicines are inadvisable for pregnant women, especially those associated with pain alleviation. To find pain relief without the use of drugs is an ideal situation and one that supports the continued health of you and your child.

There are many benefits to adding chiropractic care to your prenatal care. More and more, the benefits of prenatal chiropractic care for the health of mothers and babies is recognized by other practitioners, and their patients are seeking out licensed chiropractic professionals to help guide them through this exciting time of life.

What Should A Patient Look For In Prenatal Chiropractic?

This is an important question because not every chiropractor practices the same way! When you are searching for chiropractic care during your pregnancy, or for your child, it important to find the right kind of chiropractor for you.

All chiropractors go through an extensive amount of schooling and training, to earn their doctorate and become a Doctor of Chiropractic. However, only some chiropractors choose to specialize in specific techniques. The largest and most well-known organizing that trains chiropractors in pediatric and pregnancy care is the International Chiropractic Pediatric Association, and a database lists the doctors who have been through their training program. However, this is not the only association that offers education in this area. So, if you are interested in seeing a chiropractor and do not see them listed on the ICPA website, ask them where they received their specialty training.

Less is more! A child's spine is much more flexible than an adults. They are also constantly reaching new milestones in growth, and their bodies are constantly changing. During pregnancy your ligaments become laxer than usual due to the hormones that are being released. This is perfectly normal and necessary for preparing the body for the coming labor. So, when it comes to getting adjusted it does not take as much force as it would if you were not pregnant.

Find someone that makes you and your child comfortable. Your potential chiropractor should be someone who can engage with you at a level that you are comfortable with. They should also engage with your child in a way that makes them feel at ease, as this is especially important when it comes to working with your child.

Evaluate the office and see if it is set up to handle a patient as they go through pregnancy. There should be pregnancy pillows or a chiropractic table that has a swing-away piece, so you can lay down comfortably and safely. The office should be designed to be a safe space and designed in a way that your child can be comfortable without risking injury from equipment or other hazards. The best way to see if an office can accommodate you is to visit! Most, if not all chiropractors, would be happy to give you a tour of the office.

What Are The Benefits Of Pediatric Chiropractic?

Chiropractic care has become an effective way of addressing musculoskeletal issues and various health problems in children. According to the International Chiropractic Pediatric Association, spinal manipulative therapy is a safe way to treat kids of all ages. It is a type of healthcare without the use of drugs or invasive modalities, thus reducing the risk of side effects. Here are a few of the benefits of pediatric chiropractic:

Treating Chronic Disease in Childhood: Chronic conditions in children, such as headaches, earache, and neck pain can be effectively treated with chiropractic care. Spinal adjustments done by an expert will have a beneficial effect on the child's health and can eliminate the root cause of most chronic disease. Since the treatment is non-invasive and does not involve the use of drugs, it is a milder approach for children.

Correcting Birth Trauma: Parents often discover pediatric chiropractic care as an effective treatment for birth traumas. A child is exposed to significant stress during birth, whether the delivery is normal, performed with a C-section or is an assisted delivery (such as with forceps). Exposure to a vacuum or forceps extraction may lead to misalignment of the spine, which later develops as a chronic health condition, like allergies or chronic headaches, among others. Most acute health conditions are associated with accidental injury, encountered during birth, and can be corrected with pediatric chiropractic.

A spinal misalignment incurred during delivery may lead to various health problems later on in the child's life if left untreated. Therefore it is extremely important for any parent to visit an experienced chiropractor, to prevent further damage from developing. Here are other ways that pediatric chiropractic can benefit your child:

Improves Sleep And Behavior: If your child is experiencing difficulties sleeping for no observable reason, it may be treated effectively with a chiropractic adjustment. A chiropractor will examine your child and will remove any blockage to the neural pathways, that may be interrupted. This can help heal the nervous system and improve sleep. The technique also aids with improving circulation which, in turn, promotes relaxation and can help your child get a better quality of sleep.

Reduces Health Risks: Pediatric chiropractic care also helps reduce the risk of developing various diseases that are related to subluxations. A chiropractor may improve the overall health of your child, by preventing or delaying degenerative conditions, such as osteoporosis and osteoarthritis. It can also increase longevity and prevent your kids from losing their quality of health at an earlier age.

Why Is It So Powerful?

Parents look to chiropractic care as a complementary part of their children's health-care needs. As such, pediatric chiropractic has become one of the most utilized forms of alternative healthcare for children. Like adults, children benefit from spinal manipulation and adjustments, as well as other kinds of care that fall under the purview of chiropractic.

However, chiropractic care should work as a complementary treatment to regular pediatric care. Chiropractic care works alongside a pediatrician's treatment, but does not replace the role of a medical doctor. A pediatrician may prescribe medications for some conditions, as determined necessary, when treating a child's severe illnesses or injury. A pediatric chiropractor, on the other hand, provides preventative, supportive healthcare, as well as alternative treatment.

While it is important for adults to maintain their chiropractic care, it is extremely important that children are introduced to chiropractic care at a very young age. Even newborns can begin chiropractic care and continue it throughout their lifetime. Rapid growth and development of the spine and nervous system take place during childhood and early adolescence, which is why chiropractic care becomes so important. As a parent, it becomes essential to take charge of your child's health and have them treated, as early as possible. Pediatric chiropractic care enables your child to grow better and enjoy a high quality of life.

What Problems Can Be Addressed With Pediatric Chiropractic?

For those who suffer from aches and pains during pregnancy, chiropractic care is an advantageous option. During pregnancy, a women's body goes through many changes, and it is quite natural to experience pain in the lower to mid back, legs, among other discomforts.

Although taking painkillers may provide temporary relief from aches and pains, the baby's health is put at risk. It is an important factor to take into consideration, when seeking to manage your pain. As a substitute, most women prefer alternative medicine and name chiropractic as one of the most effective forms. This type of treatment seeks to determine the root cause of any pain and treat the underlying issue to handle the condition.

Dr. Eric Jaszewski is a member of the ICPA and is Webster-Certified and Chiropractic treatments during pregnancy, including the Webster's Technique. This technique brings balance to the pelvis area by helping the surrounding muscles and ligaments relax, as well as removing any constraints in the joints. It is essential to ensure that the pelvis is kept in good shape so that the mother and baby will be as comfortable as possible.

Massage therapy is also offered during pregnancy, which can help to de-stress the mother and improving her wellbeing. A good and gentle massage removes most discomforts that a woman may endure during pregnancy. There are many experienced practitioners who are well-trained in the latest techniques that can offer expert and comfortable care, to make pregnancy easier for the mother.

How Does Chiropractic Effect A Child's Immune System?

When it comes to chiropractic, many believe that its focus is on relieving patients' symptoms, primarily associated with musculoskeletal conditions or everyday aches and pains. However, research suggests that chiropractic intervention can also be used to boost a child's immune system.

Most parents are aware of the benefits of chiropractic care for back and neck pain. Still, a lesser-known advantage of chiropractic treatment is its ability to improve the immune system.

The nervous system affects the immune system and plays a vital role in the immune response against illness. Many factors contribute to a child's immune system's ability to maintain optimal health and combat illness, such as nutrition, exercise, posture, stress, and fatigue. These are all essential, but so is the health and condition of their spine. Misalignments of the vertebrae can put pressure on the spinal cord and nerves, which run through the length of the spine and extend out into the body. A blockage of these nerves can lead to irritation of the nervous system, and alter the ability of the it to supply tissues, organs, and cells of the with vital communications from the brain.

When it functions properly the immune system fights disease-producing organisms, such as bacteria, viruses, fungi, parasites, and allergens, all children are continuously exposed to these pathogens. Still, exposure does not automatically lead to a child becoming sick. A strong immune system provides a child with powerful natural defenses against disease. Conversely, a child with a weakened immune system is more vulnerable, and more susceptible to colds, the flu, allergies, and chronic disease.

Chiropractic adjustments can remove nerve interference, stimulate the immune system, and improve respiratory function. The immune system can then function at total capacity, allowing the body to naturally defend itself against colds and other infections.

How Does Chiropractic Effect Ear Infections?

Otitis media (OM), commonly referred to as an ear infection, is one of the most common childhood illnesses in the world. Ear infection is most commonly incurred in children up to the age of 6, and peaks around the age of 2. Unless it's treated, however, the condition can persist well into early and middle adulthood. The primary symptoms are typically are soreness, pain, and strong discomfort in the area surrounding the ear, as well as fever, fluid drainage, trouble sleeping, a loss of appetite and moody behavior.

Natural remedies and specific, gentle chiropractic adjustments have proved to be considerably effective in handling ear infections.

Hopefully, the word will spread about the advantages of chiropractic care as countless children suffer needlessly, every year.

When is dealing with an ear infection, chiropractors focus on the muscles in the neck to encourage proper function of the lymph glands within the ear. If there is a misalignment in this area of the spine, nerve function is disrupted and can hamper the process of proper drainage of the Eustachian tube in the ear. This creates a harmful buildup of bacteria and fluids, which can cause pain and the internal pressure associated with an ear infection.

Chiropractic care uses gentle manipulations and readjustments of the spine to release the internal pressure which affects the infected ear. Once a successful spinal readjustment releases the interference that was disrupting your body's proper nerve function, the Eustachian tube in the ear will begin to function correctly. So will your lymphatic vessels, and a proper, healthy drainage of fluid from the ear can then take place.

How Does Prenatal Chiropractic Specifically Affect The Mother's Well Being?

Pregnancy should be an exciting time for the coming mother and encompass many challenges for the body. Growing and carrying an unborn child puts a lot of strain and stress on a woman's body, and it is vital that she take great care of herself during this time, for her health and the health of her unborn child.

Some mothers even choose to be adjusted during labor, at the discretion of their chiropractor, doctor or midwife. Chiropractic is so safe and so important for proper health and function that even newborns can be adjusted. Chiropractic can also help the postpartum healing process, by correcting any misalignments that may have occurred during labor or birth. This ensures that the mother's body is functioning optimally, so that she can heal and nurse in good health. Chiropractic is essential for correcting posture problems and back pain which can result from breastfeeding, bottle feeding, and from carrying the baby around.

Chiropractic care is safe during pregnancy and all licensed chiropractors in pediatric chiropractic are trained to take care of a pregnant patient.

Conclusion

Regular chiropractic adjustments can help ensure a healthier and more pleasant pregnancy, labor, and birthing process. Many chiropractors are specifically trained in particular adjusting techniques for pregnant women, before, during or after labor.

Chiropractic treatment can be conducted safely throughout pregnancy. Regular chiropractic adjustments help relieve back pain, enhance nervous system performance, and offset the natal hormone distribution. For mothers desiring a drug-free, natural birth, chiropractic care can help them accomplish that goal!

CHAPTER 18

CHIROPRACTIC FOR LIFE

Chiropractic is a lifelong plan for wellness, and no condition or stage of life can go without benefiting from routine chiropractic care. Chiropractic is for infants, children, adolescents, young adults, the elderly, and many others. It is suitable for everyone: those generally in good health, as well as those suffering from various conditions or ailments.

As the body is equipped with natural, innate intelligence, it knows what its optimal state should be and how to keep itself healthy. If you are adept at maintaining your health, chiropractic can be part of a preventive healthcare routine that, if incorporated into your wellness plan, will help you stay healthier and enable you to get more out of life.

The human body is a miraculous entity! It constantly performs incredible functions, many of which we are not even conscious of on a daily level. It's on the job around the clock and executes many of its vital functions without requiring any extra effort from us. When a subluxation occurs in the spine, those blockages reduce the messages transmitted by the nerves and impair the body's ability to correct any problematic issues. Chiropractic plays a vital role in allowing innate intelligence to do its job, and regular, preventive chiropractic allows a free flow of nerve signals to all areas of the body.

Each life stage brings a different set of potential health problems and ailments; thus, even a 2-hour-old newborn can benefit from the gentle touch of a chiropractor to ensure that no misaligned vertebrae caused by the birthing process are left unhandled.

Chiropractic For Infants And Children

Childhood illnesses, such as ear infections, asthma, food allergies, and even Attention Deficit Disorder (ADD), are becoming so commonplace that many parents now accept them as a normal part of childhood. The chiropractic attitude is that the creation of human life does not automatically come with built-in problems and illnesses: it is complete and perfect until external factors alter this. One should not discount genetic factors or environmental influences since they can all impact life in different ways.

However, the average healthy baby is born well and will naturally remain healthy. Even in a world with a challenging environment, if the body is not hindered in the essential communication pathways it uses to monitor and maintain the body's optimal state.

6 FACTS THAT WILL KEEP CHILDREN HEALTHY

What if I told you six facts about the body can help you keep your child healthy? By understanding these facts, you will have the tools to remove most of the interferences that can make people unhealthy or ill.

FACT #1: The nervous system controls the functions of every cell in the body, especially the immune system. By keeping the spine in perfect order and in good condition, one can boost the immune system's strength by up to 400 percent.

FACT #2: You can eliminate many health problems when you have your child examined by someone who knows what to look for and what questions to ask as it relates to scrapes, falls, and normal childhood activities. An examination of the spine by a qualified chiropractor will help them determine if any negative changes have occurred, and corrections or adjustments can then be made to open up the way for nerve signals to operate at an optimum level.

FACT #3: Indeed, you are what you eat. Nutrition is the key to creating a strong immune system, and children must consume a varied, healthy diet that is rich in vitamins and minerals. Supplements can make up for some deficiencies, but they should not be the main source of nutrients.

FACT #4: You should aim to identify problems as they arise and seek to address their causes. A routine chiropractic examination of your child can help ensure that any subluxations are corrected before significant issues develop.

FACT #5: Leading an active lifestyle is important for a child's health. In our day and age, even children are left inactive and sedentary for hours on end, at school or home. This can lead to bad posture, poor circulation, weak bone formation, and several types of health issues in the future.

FACT # 6: Be consistent as a parent; this sets a strong example for children and is key in keeping them healthy. Start early, and continue with proper chiropractic care.

Chiropractic for Ear Infections

Ear infections can seem to be a normal part of early childhood, something considered normal for most infants. An ear infection, also called "otitis media," is an infection of the inner ear. While it is common to get an ear infection during childhood, it does not have to be a chronic childhood condition. Most young children before the age of two will incur at least one ear infection. There are more than 10 million new cases every year of ear infections, accounting for 35% of all visits to the pediatrician. It is no small matter and can lead to the pediatrician recommending surgical intervention.

Middle ear infections are caused by either a virus or a bacterial infection, which often occurs due to a build-up of fluid in the eardrum. When the fluid cannot drain from the ear, an infection may develop; thus, the objective should be to remove the liquid and avoid infection.

However, traditional medicine often seeks to handle this condition through surgery, such as the insertion of ear tubes, intended to open the ear canal and allow the fluid to drain. Notably, this is the number one surgery performed on children under two years of age.

Several problems are associated with this approach. One is that it does not always provide lasting results, and between 20% and 30% of children require the procedure to be repeated. This necessitates them being put under general anesthesia for a second time.

Even if a child does not undergo surgery, the traditional way of treating ear infections does little to help them in the long run. The primary non-surgical treatment approach is based on antibiotics. While this may treat a bacterial infection, it does nothing for viral infections but sets the child up for more infections in the future as their body becomes highly resistant to antibiotics. Antibiotics also do nothing for draining the fluid found in the ear, which is part of the initial problem.

This is where chiropractic can help! The fluid buildup caused by poor drainage often triggers an infection. If the ear canal can be opened up and surgery avoided, isn't that what would be best for the child?

Chiropractic can open up the ear canal and aid in draining the eardrum through manipulation of the C1 vertebra, which is the first cervical vertebra in the spine below the skull. This method was used by renowned chiropractor Dr. Joan Fallon from Yonkers, New York. She found that with frequent adjustments over six months, her young patients' bodies were able to drain any excess fluid from their ears on their own, resulting in an absence of ear infections!

If the child did experience an ear infection, it gave the body the information it needed to fight off future infections. By not suppressing the body's natural response and ensuring there was no blockage of the nerves in the upper cervical spine, the children developed fewer ear infections.

Chiropractic for The Treatment of Asthma

Asthma, seen to be on the rise in adults and children, has long been viewed as a condition primarily caused by genetic factors, causing the airways to become restricted due to muscle hyper-responsiveness. However, scientists, allergists, and doctors have been unable to pinpoint an exact reason for the increase in cases and have many theories about it. According to the World Health Organization, 100-150 million people worldwide are currently being treated for asthma. Much of this increase in asthmatic conditions appears to be linked to environmental causes; modern products produce more allergens and irritants are trapped in our homes and offices due to modern construction materials and insulation methods. This could explain why more cases of asthma have been diagnosed in industrialized nations.

Just about every classroom in the United States has at least one child with asthma. This can't all be hereditary;

there seem to be environmental factors that have led to an increase in asthma among American children.

Asthma has traditionally been treated with medication. The medications found in inhalers are intended to open the small bronchial passages in the lungs, allowing for a freer intake of air. These medicines are steroid-type drugs, specifically corticosteroids. Do we want our children to be inhaling steroids? Most parents would likely prefer a non-steroid approach to help their children breathe easier, as there are many side effects associated with the use of inhaled steroids. Many asthmatic children experience stunted growth in the first year they begin using an inhaler, although eventually, they return to a more regular growth pattern. Other long-term side effects include osteoporosis, hypertension, glaucoma, and diabetes — all of which are serious.

Chiropractic has been successful in treating asthma in both adults and children. There is no official cure for asthma, but treatments can provide effective relief. Acute asthma attacks may still require an inhaler, but the purpose of chiropractic is to try to remedy the cause of asthma attacks in the first place.

Some methods for preventing asthma attacks are proactive wellness techniques that go hand-in-hand with the chiropractic philosophy. These include providing a good nutritional basis for children, as when the immune system is strong and the body is well-equipped with the proper nutrients, it can correct many factors that may trigger an asthma attack. Secondly, exercise is a key factor in preventing asthma attacks for those who often suffer attacks as a result of exertion. In a sense, the child is preparing their body to handle the attack by conditioning their lungs. The instinct may be to do less activity, as activity seems to bring on the attacks; however, in reality, the opposite is true.

The goal of chiropractic in treating a child with asthma is to prevent attacks and improve the child's overall quality of life. A child who has to limit their participation in normal childhood activities will not be as happy as they could be. Thus, the goal of chiropractic is to improve the quality and quantity of activities in which the child can participate while preventing asthma attacks. No conclusive studies exist to date proving that chiropractic care can prevent attacks. However, in most practices treating children with asthma, there is evidence that the release of endorphins and other internal reactions occurring with spinal manipulation may help improve pulmonary function.

The most significant advantage of chiropractic is already known to those parents who have brought their children to the chiropractor in a last-ditch effort to find some sort of relief. Children who regularly visit the chiropractor can improve posture, which affects the mechanical function and structure of the ribs and the shoulders encasing the lungs.

Chiropractic's Counterattack on Food Allergies

Getting rid of the symptoms of food allergies can either be one of the most accessible and controllable conditions to treat or one of the most challenging conditions to treat. This dichotomy stems from either not knowing what food is causing the adverse reaction in the body or not being able to isolate the exact food or ingredient that is causing the problems.

Allergy testing for food allergies is often done by injecting a small amount of the suspected allergen into the skin and observing what happens. The substance that causes redness or swelling is identified as the cause. To treat the allergy in this case, simply remove the food from the diet; problem solved!

The difficulty arises when the allergen cannot be isolated and, therefore, cannot be removed. When infants are introduced to solid foods, parents are taught to introduce only one food at a time for several days to ensure that the baby doesn't experience any rashes, vomiting, or diarrhea. If all is well, then a new food item can be introduced. This method allows parents to observe whether any foods are not agreeable to the baby's tender system.

Chiropractic takes a similar approach to treating food allergies, or any other allergies, for that matter. Balancing out the nervous system allows the body to fight off allergies — food or otherwise. A lifestyle in which stress is under control is one in which fewer allergies will appear. Stress increases cortisol production and taxes the adrenal glands, which can then predispose the body to develop allergies. Foods laden with chemicals and additives also invite food allergies. The chiropractic way of life focuses on whole, preferably organic foods that are naturally assimilated and used by the body for good nutrition and health.

Managing ADD through Chiropractic

The diagnosis of Attention Deficit Disorder (ADD) and Attention Deficit Hyperactivity Disorder (ADHD) is growing at an alarming rate. Are there genuinely more cases, or is it that more school systems and doctors are applying this "one-size-fits-all" label to any child who is "too active", bored, has different learning needs, or is experiencing some kind of stress at home or school? These conditions are usually the underlying cause of cases misdiagnosed with ADD or ADHD.

In reality, ADD and ADHD have accompanying symptoms that go far beyond an inability to sit through a classroom period or exhibiting aggressive behavior. Those truly afflicted with the disorder usually also experience other symptoms, such as sensitivity to light, sound, and touch. They may also experience tics or tremors and suffer obvious postural problems. This last symptom is one that chiropractic best addresses, as it may also be the symptom that alleviates many of the other symptoms when treated.

Doctors of Chiropractic and, more specifically, Chiropractic Neurologists are involved with the impact that postural muscles have on brain activity. When there is a musculoskeletal imbalance, there will be an imbalance in brain activity, resulting in uneven brain development with one side of the brain surpassing the other. This is the condition associated with children who truly have Attention Deficit Disorder (ADD) or Attention Deficit Hyperactivity Disorder (ADHD).

Brain stimulation is the primary method employed by chiropractors to stimulate the development of the lagging side of the brain. This is accomplished through a series of tests that stimulate auditory and visual functions within the brain, such as flashing light or blocking light with special glasses. Auditory testing may include listening to music with only one ear. These therapies must be performed for a few months before any measurable results can be noticed.

Improving the under-functioning areas of the brain is only one step chiropractors take in treating children with ADD. They also recommend lifestyle changes that promote better nutrition and avoid the use of unnatural ingredients, such as dyes and preservatives in foods. This helps to regulate biochemical imbalances that may be contributing to a child's ADD symptoms by improving their diet in general and creating a healthier balance.

Improving a child's specific musculoskeletal imbalances and nutrition work together in treating ADD and ADHD, without the use of other medications.

Although medications may be effective in suppressing symptoms, they cease to work when they are discontinued and can often result in serious (and sometimes even life-threatening) side effects. With chiropractic methods, the changes are permanent as the brain is stimulated and allowed to develop properly.

Made in the USA
Middletown, DE
20 July 2023

35047515R00126